WELLNESS REIMAGINED

WELLNESS REIMAGINED

*A Holistic Approach to Health,
Happiness, and Harmony*

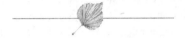

ERIN CLIFFORD
JD, MA, LPC

Forefront
BOOKS

Published by Forefront Books, Nashville, Tennessee.
Distributed by Simon & Schuster.

Library of Congress Control Number: 2025900891

Print ISBN: 978-1-63763-418-9
E-book ISBN: 978-1-63763-419-6

Cover Design by Mary Susan Oleson, Blu Design Concepts
Interior Design by Mary Susan Oleson, Blu Design Concepts

Printed in the United States of America

For my Grandma Betty,
a fearless woman
way ahead of her time.
You embodied the definition
of strength, courage,
and living a harmonious life.
You encouraged me
to believe in myself
and shoot for the stars.
I feel your presence in these pages.

CONTENTS

INTRODUCTION

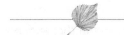

My wellness journey began when I was a child growing up in the Northwest Suburbs of Chicago. I loved running along the lake with my dad, even in winter, when snow lined the trees set against the majestic backdrop of the Chicago skyline. Though he was an extremely busy trial lawyer, my dad prioritized family and physical fitness. My mom preferred to exercise at home on the treadmill or with her Jane Fonda workout videos. I can still see those videos on our family bookshelves surrounded by lifestyle books and Tony Robbins cassettes. For fun I enjoyed riding my pink bike around our neighborhood. At night I read novels by flashlight. My parents encouraged my interests in music and theater and sports. Somehow, I balanced it all with school and community activities.

Many of my fondest childhood memories revolve

around cooking and baking with my Grandma Betty, one of my closest confidants, in our family's kitchen. She made everything from scratch, including delicious meals and desserts. Grandma Betty exercised, too, and enjoyed spending time with family and her church community. Even in her nineties she took impeccable care of herself and, to my delight, made weekly visits to her neighborhood beauty salon.

My parents and grandmother were my role models. They embodied the kind of life I wanted to achieve. They gave me confidence and motivated me to develop my own healthy routines. This served me well—to a point. In college, I became conflicted about my career and life path. During that time, I developed bulimia nervosa and an anxiety disorder. So I decided to take a semester off to get treatment. Watching friends graduate and begin living their lives, I felt like a failure. I was a perfectionist. Fortunately, I received excellent care and support from my loved ones. After college graduation, I began my teaching career. Little did I know that more challenges awaited me in the professional world.

As a Chicago Public Schools high school English teacher, I found it difficult to balance my work and personal lives. I loved teaching, but I felt uncertain about what I valued and wanted for my life. My confidence faded. Chronic stress and burnout reached a boiling point, leading to a relapse of my eating disorder. After another period of treatment, I resolved to make a big change. I decided to go to law school. I moved to the city with Bella, my Bernese mountain dog. That decision completely changed and saved my life.

When I began my law career, I clerked on the Illinois Appellate Court for an amazing judge. That's where I connected with three of my closest girlfriends. I loved being a part of the legal community and felt blessed to ultimately work with my dad at our family's law firm. I also learned firsthand the inherent stressors of the profession. From experience, I knew that my own well-being needed to come first. That's when I began to explore my own wellness on a deeper level and create a more harmonious, values-based lifestyle. Wellness, I discovered, wasn't just a way of life. It became my calling. My purpose. My heart would break when I saw my colleagues and friends struggle. I wanted to share with them what I was learning about wellness.

This inspired me to become certified as a health and wellness coach through the Institute for Integrative Nutrition. I continued to educate myself on all things wellness, connecting with leading practitioners and earning more coaching certifications in lifestyle areas of nutrition, mindfulness, self-care, stress management, sleep hygiene, and physical fitness. I expanded my business and began to work with professionals, law firms, and corporations. I was learning that wellness is holistic. Physical, mental, emotional, and spiritual well-being are all intertwined. So I went back to school at Northwestern University and attained a master's degree in mental health counseling. My clinical internship was with an excellent treatment center in Chicago dedicated to helping professionals struggling with substance misuse and addiction. I now consider myself in recovery too.

Turns out I *am* a teacher—just not in the sense I originally planned as a young person. Nothing brings me greater joy than sharing my expertise with others. Work and life are stressful. Some periods are more difficult than others. I've learned there is no such thing as perfect balance. Harmony, however, is more than possible. It's possible to establish and maintain a healthy, happy, and harmonious life. That's what I want to share with you.

My intention in writing this book is to empower you to live life on your own terms.

You can custom-make a life that brings you

optimum fulfillment and satisfaction. This book is your invitation to pause in your busy life and decide how you want to live—and empower yourself to live it.

WHAT IS WELLNESS?

Often the word *wellness* is used in contrast with *illness*. If one is well, they aren't sick. But wellness is not just the absence of disease. It's about the *presence* of life in body, mind, and soul. It's physical, mental, emotional, and spiritual well-being.

As individuals progress through the different stages of life, their wants, needs, and values shift. Wellness ebbs and flows like the rhythm of the ocean tides. Both positive and negative experiences impact wellness. Wellness, therefore, is highly individualized. It looks different for each person.

My clients reach out to me with wildly different motivations, holding unique reasons for wanting to make lifestyle shifts. They are often seeking ways to illuminate their wellness, whether it be in their body, mind, or soul. Katie received a chronic disease diagnosis and needed assistance reshaping her routines for self-care. She wanted to be healthy for her children and grandchildren. Bill transitioned from a high-stress career into retirement and wanted to revamp his next act to enjoy the fruits of his labor. Christine wrestled with finding balance between her high-powered career and life as a mother. You, too, have a unique why for wanting to make lifestyle changes.

Many high-performing professionals struggle with unattainable standards. I recognize the all-or-nothing belief because I used to share it. Perfectionism contributes to workplace stress and burnout.[1] It also leads to isolation and robs us of genuine connection with others. Perfectionism may even lead to the abandonment of wellness pursuits altogether. A cornerstone of wellness, in my view, is that *something is always better than nothing.* It's about the big picture, not a single day, week, or month.

Adaptation is key to wellness. I recently met a new father, Matt, during a corporate workshop. Matt had completely abandoned his exercise routine because his new schedule did not allow him to work out at his former intensity. He'd struggled to accept shorter workouts. I urged Matt to find pockets of time for self-care rather than giving up. Doing so required a shift toward a self-compassionate lens.

It's not just about compassion; it's also about productivity. A cultural shift is currently happening in America.

Introduction

As rates of chronic diseases have continued to rise over the past decade, health-care costs have increased dramatically. Research suggests that 80 percent of chronic diseases are completely preventable with healthy food and lifestyle choices.[2] Stress alone costs American business $300 billion each year and contributes to absenteeism and low productivity, according to the World Health Organization. As such, many corporations are ramping up employee wellness programs with benefits such as gym memberships, health workshops, office challenges, and hybrid schedules.

While this trend toward workplace wellness initiatives appears promising, working professionals need real solutions that align with their go-go-go lives. Wellness needs to be achievable and doable. Strategizing comes into play here. Lifestyle changes work best when individuals are empowered with realistic, sustainable solutions that bring more positivity and productivity to their lives.

Inspiration for this can be found in one of my favorite books. In Lewis Carroll's *Alice's Adventures in Wonderland*, Alice comes to a fork in the road. There she asks the Cheshire Cat which way she "ought to go" but has no understanding of where she wants to get to in her journey. The Cat wisely notes, "Then it doesn't matter which way you go."

You may be at a metaphorical fork in the road. But unlike Alice, you want to go someplace. It *does* matter which way you go. This book will give you the necessary tools to choose your desired path.

The first step will involve a little self-reflection. You'll need to get quiet and ask yourself some questions and then answer them honestly. You'll discover your why, which will guide the development of your lifestyle plan. Through this journey you will:

- Reflect on your current values system to discover what life domains need shifting.

- Learn to create personal and professional boundaries.

- Set daily routines that are flexible and meet individual needs.

- Explore areas of self-care, including exercise, nutrition, mindful stress management, and sleep hygiene.

- Discover strategies to troubleshoot and maintain wellness routines during busy seasons.

- Set SMART goals that align with values-based harmonious living to achieve personal and professional success.

Introduction

As a childhood fan of the Choose Your Own Adventure book series, I intentionally created this program to be unique to you. My own experience has taught me that no one path to wellness exists. Consider this guide a choose-your-own wellness adventure and create a plan authentic to you.

FOREWORD

IN TODAY'S FAST-PACED, success-driven world, where wellness is often reduced to fleeting trends or recommendations that don't cater to the realities of life, *Wellness Reimagined: A Holistic Approach to Health, Happiness, and Harmony* offers something transformative—a realistic, customizable, and truly sustainable guide to wellness. Erin Clifford has created more than a wellness solution; she's crafted a resource for self-discovery, purpose, and growth. For professionals seeking not only to thrive in their careers but to live in alignment with their deepest values, this book is an invitation to breathe easier, find renewed energy, and build a life that is both successful and fulfilling. With Erin as your compassionate, insightful coach, *Wellness Reimagined* is the perfect companion to embrace wellness as an essential part of your life.

Erin Clifford is uniquely qualified to lead you on this journey, drawing from her own experience in high-stress environments and extensive background in education and wellness work. While she wears many hats in life, including managing director at her family law firm, corporate wellness consultant, speaker, board member, wife, devoted family member, and friend, I'd also like to add inspiration. While wellness has always been part of my company's core values, Erin's wellness wisdom took us to new levels. As my team and I supported Erin with design, we'd get what I called "fire-y and inspire-y," learning from her while we created her educational assets. Her inspiration ignited action throughout my company as we all made healthy changes, additions, or adaptations. I'm so thankful for the ways Erin has elevated my wellness personally, and as an employer, I'm beyond grateful for how she helped power up my company's positivity and productivity. I'll never forget sitting with Erin at her dining room table in Chicago. She had made time to see me when I was in town, even as she was in the thick of writing her thesis for her master's in mental health from Northwestern University. As our dogs played, we caught up over tea talking about life, work, and goals. Her number one nonnegotiable must-do was to bring her decades of wellness expertise together into a book to help more people claim wellness that works. It gives me great joy to see this dream become a reality, knowing how many lives Erin will enhance with this beautiful book.

Wellness isn't a luxury or an extra task on the to-do list; it's an essential foundation for success, productivity, and satisfaction, both personally and professionally. Erin Clifford understands that wellness isn't about an idealized notion of balance but about creating harmony, giving us a foundation to thrive among life's various domains: career, relationships, physical health, mental resilience, and personal fulfillment. This is a resource for life—now, in the future, and generationally. Whether you're taking your first step toward wellness or refining a well-traveled path, *Wellness Reimagined* equips you with tools to adapt, grow, and thrive. Erin reminds us that wellness isn't a fixed destination—it's an ongoing relationship with yourself, evolving alongside your needs and goals.

Get ready to embark on your ideal wellness journey with your new personal wellness GPS system!

Lorrie Thomas Ross
CEO AND THE MARKETING THERAPIST®
WEB MARKETING THERAPY INC.

PART I

HARMONIOUS LIVING

1 IDENTIFY YOUR PERSONAL VALUES

*When your values are clear to you,
making decisions becomes easier.*

—Roy E. Disney

VALUES ARE THE fundamental beliefs that govern an individual's life. Each person lives according to a unique set of values based on life experiences. Values necessarily shift and evolve over time. They serve as our North Star and point us in the direction of the life we want to live. Values represent the things that are most important to us. They also embody a central part of who we are and who we want to become. Research has found that when individuals live in accordance with their values, it creates higher psychological well-being.[3] This value congruence produces greater life satisfaction, self-esteem, and positive affect, and it reduces internal conflicts. Research also suggests that values may be used to guide behavioral change and allow individuals to produce the outcomes they most desire.[4] As such, when you are clear about your values, you can more easily make meaningful decisions in your life domains.

When an individual's values do not align with decisions and actions, it creates disharmony and contributes to chronic stress. After all, it's challenging to live the life you want when you're constantly running in the opposite direction of your values. While you might be able to manage it for a period or even years, it will eventually lead to burnout and feeling unfulfilled. For example, my client Tom valued family, yet he created a daily life that afforded him little time at home. This disconnect caused increasing dissatisfaction with his life. Mariah valued her health. But her work stress caused her to disengage from her self-care practices and she developed a chronic illness. Fred valued his spirituality and struggled with depression when he moved away from his longtime church community.

Reflecting on my core values played a prominent role in recovering from challenging times. I learned to use my values to make intentional decisions and build a fulfilling life. I was often painfully hard on myself. I felt pressured to earn high marks in school and then find the perfect job. I struggled with my body image and society's ever-changing unrealistic expectations for women. *Grace* emerged as a high value for me. It now serves as my compass and has led me toward a life of self-compassion. Yes, I still have my critical moments. But I am always able to take a breath and give myself grace.

My values also guided me as I developed in my career. *Freedom* became extremely important to me, and I created a daily life that afforded me more flexibility. While I enjoy going into the office to connect with clients and colleagues, I can also work remotely when necessary. I discovered that I thrive when I have more control over my daily schedule. Further, I strive to show up in the world with *authenticity*. It's a hallmark of how I interact with my clients and during presentations. I am a much better human being and coach when I stay true to who I am.

Additionally, I strive for *harmony* in my life domains and lifestyle routine. To be at my best I need to feel like my personal and professional spaces are coexisting, even if I may be more focused in one domain than the other. I no longer have an all-or-nothing mentality. I balance my self-care and celebrate little wins. For example, I eat a balanced diet and don't deny myself foods that I enjoy in moderation. I also listen to what my body needs related to physical fitness. Sometimes it's better to stretch and go in the sauna for recovery as opposed to doing another challenging workout.

One value that has never wavered for me is *family*. My close-knit family (and friends whom I consider family) will always be my number one priority. I love nothing more than spending time with my people who bring so much joy to my life. It has been such a gift to work at our family's law firm with my father, cousins, and husband. I love spending time with my mom and sister. We never miss our annual Christmas tea at the Peninsula Hotel. And nothing makes me smile more than my nephews and dogs. I prioritize communicating with my friends and getting the ladies together for pizza night. After all, even when life gets busy it's important to stay connected to those you value most.

As you begin to reflect on your own core values, consider how they were shaped. Childhood environments often influence an individual's early values system. Kevin, whose family valued hard work, felt driven to excel in school and athletics. Karen's family raised her in a religious community where spirituality and philanthropic endeavors mattered most. The internal workings of family also contribute to how human beings view relationships. For example, Elliot's parents divorced when he was a child. As a result, he strived to create a strong nuclear family with his wife. When personal beliefs become incongruent with those of family and friends, it can be challenging. When Kiara married a man outside her faith it created strife among her family and childhood friends. Caleb also experienced familial disappointment when he pursued his passion of becoming a high school science teacher as opposed to going to medical school.

Further, values and priorities change as individuals progress through life stages and develop identities. Young professionals may hold very different beliefs than their colleagues deep into their careers or nearing retirement. For example, when Charlie began his career, he regularly traveled to national conferences to build his business. At the peak of her career, Jana became president of her local women's bar association. Whereas Sam transitioned into semi-retirement by mentoring young talent. When I got married my priorities shifted and opened a whole new way of living. Decisions were not just about me. For years I'd enjoyed networking late into the evening. Now I crave lazy nights at home, cooking dinner with my husband, John.

Cultural norms also have evolved over the years. Society is not the determining factor for when individuals might choose to marry, start families, or pursue career opportunities. My client Beth went back to graduate school and began a new career in counseling when her children left for college. Lucas and his partner adopted a child and fulfilled their dream of becoming parents. Chloe left her financially lucrative position at a Fortune 500 company to run a nonprofit for a cause that she personally championed. It's up to you to determine your values and how you should live your life.

As you begin this wellness journey, start by recognizing where your focus truly lies right now by engaging with your current values system. What does success look like to you personally and professionally? Consider both your positive and negative experiences. Each event gives you data. Think about times and occurrences that energized you, brought you joy, made you feel fulfilled, or made you most proud. Also consider situations that extinguished your spark, brought you distress, or made you feel uncomfortable or incongruent to your authentic self. Do you have any cultural or community considerations that are important to you? Humans have a limited amount of time on this earth. Spend it your way and with the people who bring you the most fulfillment.

VALUES REFLECTION

This reflection allows you space to become crystal clear about your top five values. Determine what your values mean to you, and they will serve as a North Star for your lifestyle plan development. These core values will also become your guide for making life decisions and building a more authentic and purposeful future.

Below is a list of values. As you complete this section, follow these steps:

1. Examine the list of values and cross off half of them that don't apply to you.

2. Go through the remaining list of values and circle your top ten.

3. Consider your top ten values and select your top five.

Review the Following List of Values:

Accountability	Efficiency	Intuition	Responsibility
Achievement	Equality	Job security	Risk taking
Adaptability	Ethics	Joy	Safety
Adventure	Excellence	Justice	Security
Altruism	Fairness	Kindness	Self-discipline
Ambition	Faith	Knowledge	Self-expression
Authenticity	Family	Leadership	Self-respect
Balance	Financial stability	Learning	Serenity
Beauty	Forgiveness	Legacy	Service
Being the best	Freedom	Leisure	Simplicity
Belonging	Friendship	Love	Spirituality
Career	Fun	Loyalty	Sportsmanship
Caring	Future generations	Making a difference	Stewardship
Collaboration	Generosity	Nature	Success
Commitment	Giving back	Openness	Teamwork
Community	Grace	Optimism	Thrift
Compassion	Gratitude	Order	Time
Competence	Growth	Parenting	Tradition
Confidence	Harmony	Patience	Travel
Connection	Health	Patriotism	Trust | Truth
Contentment	Home	Peace	Uniqueness
Contribution	Honesty	Perseverance	Usefulness
Cooperation	Hope	Personal fulfillment	Vision
Courage	Humility	Power	Vulnerability
Creativity	Humor	Pride	Wealth
Curiosity	Inclusion	Recognition	Well-being
Dignity	Independence	Reliability	Wholeheartedness
Diversity	Initiative	Resourcefulness	Wisdom
Environment	Integrity	Respect	

Record your top five values and explain what each value means to you.

1. _____

_____

_____

2. _____

_____

_____

3. _____

_____

_____

4. _____

_____

_____

5. _____

_____

_____

_____

_____

Reflection

How did you experience this exercise? Was it easy or difficult? Did you have to do any negotiating to narrow down your values? _____

_____

_____

_____

How have your values shifted over time? _____

_____

_____

Do you feel like you are living according to your values in your personal and professional lives? Why or why not?

_____

_____

_____

Do you recognize life domains (i.e., career, family, health, spirituality) that need attention to be more aligned with your values? _____

_____

_____

_____

VALUES CHALLENGE

For the next five weeks choose one of your top values to focus on each week. Be mindful of how your daily actions, words, and decisions reflect your chosen value. Hold yourself accountable by displaying your weekly value on a Post-it Note somewhere that is visible. You may also choose to tell a loved one about your challenge. Keep a daily journal to reflect on your progress. Each night record some thoughts about how successful you were in living your value. Document any wins and note any hurdles that you might have encountered. Over time this practice will allow you to automatically weave your values into daily living and will guide you in making choices that align with the person you want to be.

2 | WORK-LIFE HARMONY

You can do anything, but not everything.

—DAVID ALLEN

WHEN I WAS little my dad took my sister and me to the Barnum and Bailey circus. I watched in awe as acrobats in sparkling costumes walked across the tightrope suspended high above us. I wondered, *What if they fall?* With a misplaced foot, they might stumble and fall on top of us. It was fascinating and terrifying. The word *balance* conjures this impossible image in my mind. To balance means to evenly distribute weight. By implication this makes me think of scales and percentage points. Today the task of balancing life often adds anxiety and stress.

Though circus acts thrilled me as a child, music gave me joy. When harmonizing with my fellow actors and in the church choir, my unique voice came alongside other voices—and the result was beautiful. Harmony happens when differing notes sound at the same time with a pleasing effect. Visual artists use harmony too, creating compositions by blending shapes, tones, or textures in gratifying ways. I employ the word *harmony* to similar effect when it comes to life. Instead of trying for balance, what if we tried for harmony?

Work-life harmony means intentionally crafting life domains in a way that brings the most life satisfaction. It allows for weaving life domains together so an individual can live a more intentional and fulfilling life. All the necessary domains remain present and spin together in what I call a *wheel of harmony*.

Life domains often overlap. The key is to craft the overlaps with intention for maximum life satisfaction. Chris, for instance, serves on a philanthropic hospital board he's passionate about and does so with friends with whom he desires to cultivate greater relationship. Tiffany coaches her son's soccer team, creating more family time as well as a connection to her community. Jeff trains at a local gym to enhance his self-care and connect with a social support network. Jane joined a local bar organization where she enriches her professional development and forms new relationships with colleagues. By intentionally connecting domains, pursuits that could otherwise be difficult to balance create harmony, leading to greater fulfillment.

Human beings also go through different seasons in life where some domains take center stage and others move to the background. Values often dictate these shifts. As a young professional, Steve focused on building his client portfolio, finances, and professional development. As he neared retirement, his focus shifted to personal development, spirituality, and contribution even as he continued his career.

Your unique wheel of harmony should reflect your values and goals at this stage in your life. Like a spider intentionally weaves her unique web, you will be doing the same. Start by considering the following life domains. Be intentional about what brings you the most fulfillment as you move through the different stages of life.

LIFE DOMAINS

Career

The concept of career and work can hold diverse meanings for different individuals. For instance, Ben views career as a necessary mechanism to provide for his lifestyle. He works a satisfactory job that provides a reasonable salary, health insurance, and a flexible schedule that affords him ample time to spend with his family. On the other hand, Beth views her role as a doctor as an integral part of her identity. She's passionate about helping her patients and mentoring residents. Different life stages influence career. Consider what career means to you at this moment in your life and how it impacts your other life domains.

Finance

Finances and financial stress can have a big influence on an individual's overall mental and physical health. It also determines access to opportunities in life. This domain may be intrinsically linked to the career domain. Further, unexpected life challenges may play a role in financial stability (i.e., illness, divorce, inflation). Individual expectations differ on what it means to be financially solvent or successful. Again, life stages play a part in the importance of finances.

Family and Friends

From a wellness and values perspective, healthy relationships with friends and family yield big benefits. As I always tell my clients, *money and success cannot hug you back*. It's important to maintain boundaries, prioritize downtime, and communicate with people you love in healthy ways.

Community

In blue zones, areas of the world where people consistently live for over one hundred years, researchers have noted a common theme: community.[5] Human beings are social creatures. Connection with others fosters well-being. Isolation, by contrast, leads to feeling mentally, emotionally, spiritually, and physically unwell. Find communities that give you a sense of belonging, whether it be a church, neighborhood, school, recovery group, health club, social club, or professional association. Community also often serves as a bridge, connecting other life domains. Being part of a community also means accountability. Others are there to ask if you're okay. Which leads us to the next domain.

Health

Health is wealth. Without it, the other life domains suffer. Prioritize physical and mental well-being in your wheel of harmony. Make time for preventative medical appointments (i.e., annual physical, dental cleaning, mammogram, colonoscopy) and immediately seek treatment for any health issues that arise. Professionals who work in high-stress jobs may also be at risk for developing mental health issues including depression, anxiety, and substance misuse. In fact, current research suggests that psychological disorders are increasing at an alarming rate.[6] Be attentive and notice and address any signs of chronic stress and burnout.

Self-Care

Self-care means engaging in activities that promote joy and incorporate positive supports into daily routines. Self-care aims to increase mental and physical well-being. Areas include prioritizing sleep hygiene, exercise, and healthy food choices; practicing mindfulness; using vacation time; maintaining healthy boundaries; and engaging in hobbies. Even during busy times, lean into the philosophy that something is better than nothing. Make time for smaller pockets of self-care. For instance, you may get too busy for your planned hour-long workout, but you can do ten minutes of desk exercises or go for a short walk during an afternoon snack break.

Personal Development

Change is the only constant in life. As we age, continuing to learn and grow leads to greater personal fulfillment. Take a class, learn a hobby, travel, form new relationships, or change up physical environments to challenge stagnation. The brain stays sharp, literally forming new neural pathways, when presented with new information, events, and experiences.[7]

Spirituality

Spirituality means different things to different individuals. It generally encompasses belief in something greater than the self. For some, this looks like the practice of religion or a belief in a higher power. Others may experience it in nature or in connection to other living souls. Consider exploring your spiritual well-being through avenues such as church services, meditation, prayer, nature, recovery community, music, art, and practicing gratitude.

Contribution

Investing time, love, and energy into others positively impacts overall well-being and gives life meaning. Investments look like serving on philanthropic boards, volunteering for personal causes, advocating for change in communities, coaching teams, and mentoring others. In fact, psychoanalyst Erik Erikson believed that when human beings contributed to future generations, they gained higher life satisfaction and left behind a legacy.[8] Consider how you pay it forward in the world.

Attitude

Attitude greatly affects overall wellness. Optimism contributes to increased happiness, health, and decreased negative outcomes throughout life, whereas pessimism leads to decreased wellness overall.[9] In my own life, I employ gratitude practices to bolster wellness and calm anxious thoughts. For example, each morning I reflect on five things that I am grateful for and set a positive intention for the day. I also engage in this practice right before a speaking engagement. It focuses my mind and allows me to authentically connect with my audience. Some of my clients engage in meditation, listen to podcasts, and read self-help books to increase optimism. Ultimately, a positive attitude leads to greater harmony in life.

WHEEL OF HARMONY
REFLECTION

Draw your current wheel of harmony. Circle the number that best corresponds to how satisfied you are with each life domain. When you have assessed each domain, connect the circles to create a holistic picture of your overall work-life harmony. With the insight into whether your life is providing you with the necessary harmony to meet your individual needs and goals, you may decide to make some adjustments toward greater harmony.

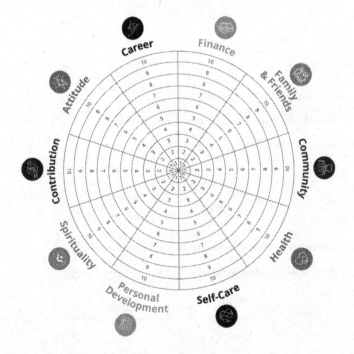

Does what you've recorded here accurately reflect your needs, priorities, and values? _____

_____

_____

Which domains currently bring you the greatest life satisfaction? _____

_____

_____

Where do you see your life domains overlap?

_____

_____

_____

Which domains would you like to improve to increase your overall life satisfaction? _____

_____

_____

What is one small step you can take immediately to shift your overall life satisfaction and prioritize your values?

_____

_____

Draw Your Inspirational Wheel

Now using a different color, draw what you desire your wheel of harmony to look like moving forward. Start by choosing *three* slices of the wheel that you'd like to invest more in. Dream a little about what you might enjoy in each of those three categories. (For instance, Self-care: meditation, massages, teeth whitening. Personal development: learn a new language.) Get creative. Follow your intuition about where you might grow next. This will allow you to bring more focus to your top life domains by weaving them together to produce more harmony.

Connect Your Values

Write a paragraph using each one of your top five values expressing how each will influence your life domains going forward. _____

_____

_____

_____

_____

CLIENT EXAMPLE—JENNY

Jenny, at forty-two, wants to make equity partner at her law firm by age fifty. Married to her college sweetheart, she has two children, ages twelve and fourteen. Trying to balance her personal and professional lives is tough. A recent diagnosis of prediabetes at her last physical exam indicates a need for a lifestyle change to accommodate self-care. Jenny's biggest motivation for change is her family.

Jenny's Highest Values: Career, Harmony, Family, Well-Being, Grace

Jenny's Inspirational Wheel of Harmony—Domains of Focus: Career, Finances, Family and Friends, Health, Self-Care, Attitude

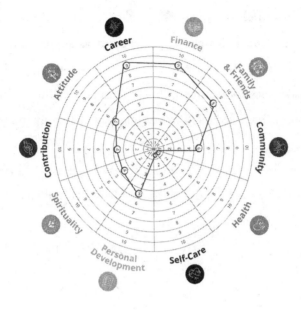

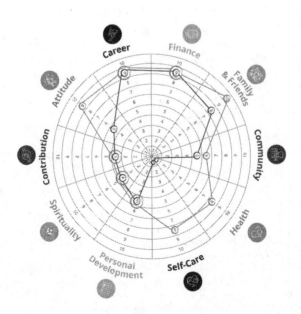

Jenny's Values Paragraph

I am focused on working diligently to achieve my career goals. I am also committed to my own well-being. I will make my self-care a top priority so I can be healthy for my family. I am dedicated to creating more harmony in my life and enjoying precious time with my children. I know there will be challenges along the way. I will handle them by shifting my mindset to give myself grace and take life a day at a time.

3 CREATE A PERSONAL BOUNDARIES POLICY

Boundaries are like fences;
they keep out what you don't want
and protect what you value.

—Henry Cloud

It can be easy when juggling responsibilities to forget our agency—that is, we have the right to say yes as well as no. I advise my clients to take a personal inventory of physical and emotional cues that may indicate permeable personal boundaries.

I have a confession: I struggle with my boundaries. For years I didn't know how or when to set them. Early in my career, my colleagues Kim and Marya gifted me a red "NO" button that voiced ten versions of no. They'd noticed I had a hard time saying no and wanted to help me out. That served as a big wake-up call for me. My girl-friends at work had observed my struggles. Now I regularly check in on my boundaries.

Boundaries are limits and rules we set and maintain in life, the workplace, and in relationships. Intentional boundaries help prioritize personal wellness. Boundaries protect our priorities. Setting boundaries also leads to better time management, increased productivity, and a reduction of overall stress.[10] There is no need to feel guilty about setting them. Boundaries are a necessary tool to navigate personal and professional spaces.

Creating a personal boundaries policy requires mindfulness. It means being intentional about how specific circumstances impact our body, mind, and spirit. What you want and what you need are a choice you must make—otherwise someone or something will choose for you. Without boundaries, you may suffer burnout. For instance, Craig, physically exhausted after a few busy weeks at work, accepted his friend's Saturday night dinner invitation out of guilt. Though Craig desperately needed a quiet evening at home, he went out and was too tired to enjoy it.

Further, boundaries help us make decisions that align with our values. When Sarah decided to focus more on her family domain, she saw that time boundaries disallowed her joining a charity board. Purchasing tickets to their annual fundraiser, however, and donating an auction item to that charity cost her little to no family time. She also noted that a no *now* does not mean a no indefinitely. When her time obligations loosen up in a few years, she will revisit the board request.

Saying yes to responsibilities takes up mental space and weight in addition to the time and resources they demand. Listening to emotions may help influence boundary setting. Consider specific requests and scan your body to see if those requests make you feel anxious, overwhelmed, unsafe, depressed, happy, or excited. Determining how the request makes you feel will help you decide if you should push the yes or no button.

Communicate your healthy boundaries. Set limits without ambiguity and assert them as needed. You are not obligated to provide a detailed explanation. Less is more. Some people will not like it when you set boundaries. That's okay.

Finally, flexibility is key. Porous boundaries may cause chronic stress. Imagine a colander where all the water drains out—that's what it looks like when you don't have good boundaries. On the other hand, rigid boundaries keep out stress but may create isolation. Stay flexible to keep healthy boundaries and recognize your own right to enforce them—or relax them.

Review the following categories. Consider where you may need new or better boundaries to create a more harmonious life.

Time Boundaries

Trying to meet others' needs can lead to overwhelm. When overcommitted, we're likely to underdeliver, both at home and at work. Setting time boundaries can help individuals avoid taking on too much. For example, Jim designates Sunday as his family day and chooses to decline all social invitations for Sundays. At work, Lindsey considers how long a project will take to complete so she can plan her schedule accordingly. This also saves her the added stress of overpromising to her superiors.

Self-Care Boundaries

Professionals often allow work and social obligations to get in the way of nourishing their self-care domain (i.e., exercise, mindfulness, sleep, meal prep, therapy, etc.). When self-care gets sidelined, burnout and unmanageability follow. Building self-care into daily and weekly routines makes it more doable and achievable. For instance, Steph often says no to weeknight after-work events so she can get her sleep in and consistently make her morning workout sessions.

Technology Boundaries

Technology plays a huge role in professional and personal lives. It seems to have become a blessing and a curse. Too much technology—calls, emails, texts, social media, apps, streaming services—can make a person feel anxious, stressed, and/or depressed. Some think they need to respond immediately to emails and texts. This may promote ill-informed decision-making. Further, social media often causes individuals to compare themselves to others, which can wreak havoc on mental and emotional health. Technological boundaries include:

- Time limits for certain social media apps

- Set breaks from social media apps altogether

- Using "Do not disturb" while working or doing other important tasks

- Committing to a no-screen policy during meals

- Not checking or answering work emails at the end of the workday

Social Boundaries

FOMO (fear of missing out) can be tough to overcome. However, before saying yes to invitations, consider if going to this event will disrupt other things that are of more importance, such as meeting a work deadline, sticking to a bedtime routine, or having dinner at home with the family. Creating social boundaries may be as simple as determining how many social obligations feel doable per month. Remember, a true friend will always grant a rain check.

Emotional Boundaries

Emotional boundaries protect an individual's emotional energy. Taking on other people's negative emotions becomes exhausting. When people set emotional boundaries, they draw a clear line of what is and is not acceptable. For example, Paul's colleague often uses him as a sounding board for office gossip. When setting emotional boundaries, Paul needed to politely communicate that he did not feel comfortable with that direction in conversation and then pivoted to a more neutral topic.

Relationship Boundaries

Healthy relationships allow individuals to consistently surround themselves with people who uplift their spirits.

Earlier we discussed how values shift over time—so, too, do relationships. Human beings sometimes outgrow relationships that used to fit well. Be sure to invest time and energy in people who bring value to your life. Joe needed to move on from some relationships that no longer served him in his sobriety. Whether it's a family member or an old friend from high school, there's no excuse for bad behavior.

Further, partnerships with significant others require clear communication to be successful long-term. After all, when partners fight about the garbage disposal not working, the appliance is probably not what they're really fighting about. It can be helpful to plan out what to say before entering a difficult or uncomfortable conversation. A note can even be sent as a prerequisite to set up the discussion. You can always circle back if you need time to think about something or regret speaking harshly.

Material Boundaries

Material boundaries allow individuals to set limits and not overextend their wallets. The finance domain gives people a sense of security and may greatly impact familial relationships, even influencing life decisions. In this day of technology, it can also be easy to overspend. My husband often comments on the number of Amazon boxes that arrive at our home each week with my name on them. Lack of boundaries with money or possessions when lending to friends or colleagues may create resentment, especially if they do not pay you back or return the item. Conversely, being too tight with finances and resources can mean missing out on enjoying hard-earned success. Most people will never regret an amazing vacation or experience.

Professional Boundaries

Setting professional boundaries with colleagues or in an office setting can be complicated. Work brings out many stressors. It can be difficult to know when to speak up while respecting the chain of command. Here are five strategies to establish healthy boundaries in the workplace:

- *Be a clear communicator.* It's perfectly acceptable to ask questions if something seems unclear or needs clarification. Respond directly and honestly in verbal and written communications. Being straightforward will establish boundaries about intentions and will leave no room for misinterpretation.

- *Learn how to delegate.* You do not need to do everything. In fact, many professional environments thrive on teamwork. Knowing strengths and weaknesses in the workplace allows individuals to say yes to some projects while saying no to others. Don't be afraid to ask for additional help or resources.

- *Identify nonnegotiables.* Stick to nonnegotiables. If exercise during the workday is a must, schedule it as if it were any other appointment. Plan work meetings around it and reschedule it immediately if necessary. Set clear hours for nonemergency work emails or calls in the evenings and include work hours in the email signage. If an individual needs to work overtime, they should ask about monetary or PTO compensation.

- *Know daily energy and workflow.* Human beings all have different energy patterns. Think of the morning person and the night owl. When possible, individuals should schedule meetings and engage in larger tasks when they are feeling more energized. Alternatively, when the battery is running low, individuals should catch up on smaller tasks like returning emails or paperwork. Also, it can be helpful to create clear structure during the workday (i.e., routines) and be mindful of others' time (i.e., structured meeting agendas).

- *Differentiate between work and nonwork activities.* The rise in working from home and technological advancements has blurred the boundaries between work and nonwork for many individuals.[11] Yet research indicates that this culture leads to professionals experiencing more exhaustion, burnout, and less work-life balance.[12] Therefore, give yourself breaks in your daily routine for self-care. Also, appreciate that you are entitled to step away from your phone and computer to enjoy living a fulfilling life and connecting with others.

BOUNDARIES REFLECTION

Spend some time reflecting on your boundaries. Answer the following questions and complete the boundaries chart below. Consider each category and determine if you need to set any boundaries to be more aligned with your wheel of harmony. Use the chart as a reference for future SMART goal setting.

What physical cues let you know that you need to set or reinforce your boundaries (i.e., GI discomfort, feelings of exhaustion, rapid heartbeat, tightness in chest)?

_____

_____

_____

_____

What emotional cues let you know that you need to set or reinforce your boundaries (i.e., discomfort, resentment, guilt, anxiety)? _____

_____

_____

_____

What is one boundary that you need to create in each area to feel more aligned with your values and wheel of harmony? Set one now and one you'd like to establish in the coming months/year. _____

_____

_____

_____

_____

Time Boundary	
Self-Care Boundary	
Technology Boundary	
Social Boundary	
Emotional Boundary	
Relationship Boundary	
Material Boundary	
Professional Boundary	

PART II

SELF-CARE ROUTINES

4 | OXYGEN
MASK RULE

You can't really be present
for the people in your life
if you aren't taking care of yourself.

—KERRY WASHINGTON

I USED TO WEAR "self-care" as a badge of honor, like a martyr. I'd complain, "I barely had time to run six miles this morning." If I had a project due at 2 p.m., I'd work through lunch. Then I'd hurry to grab a gift on the way to after-work events only to have three cocktails and later fall asleep with my makeup on.

My own self-care has evolved over the years. It's no longer punishing—too much exercise, strict diet, crammed social life—but instead it's nourishing and joyful. I love to grocery shop, cook, read in bookstores, travel, and connect with animals. I even took my mom to the Shedd Aquarium to get in the water with a beluga whale. That's self-care! Yes, it's still about adding healthy lifestyle initiatives like exercise, nutrition, mindful stress management, and sleep hygiene. But we can pack only so much in. Intention is the key. We need to make time for the smaller things that bring joy. As my mom always says, it's the little things that make for a happy life.

Self-care is about incorporating support into your routines to increase your mental, emotional, physical, and spiritual well-being.[13] We all know life may get in the way, leading to interruptions in self-care. When this occurs, self-care is often delayed or abandoned altogether. Individuals may even feel guilty about self-care. But self-care is not about being selfish. It's actually essential.

We neglect self-care to our own detriment and the detriment of others. I refer to this as the oxygen mask rule. You've likely heard flight attendants share some variation of the following: "Should the cabin lose pressure, oxygen masks will drop from the overhead area. Please *place the mask over your own mouth and nose first before assisting others.*" Why? Because if you cannot breathe, you cannot help others. The principle applies in all areas of life. You can't help others unless you yourself are healthy.

We each have a unique set of personal needs (beyond the basic survival needs) that must be met for us to be at our best.[14] Personal needs are unique to you. They are critical for you to thrive and live a life you love. They also enhance the quality of your relationships. We can meet them in both positive and negative ways. For instance, if Noah needs to feel a sense of belonging, he may choose to join a professional organization or may overcommit to social events. When Camie craves intimacy, she may choose to spend time with her partner or emotionally eat. If Terran needs to feel relaxed after a stressful day at work, he can take a yoga class or drink a bottle of wine. It's really about that underlying feeling that you are trying to create or soothe. Therefore, when you develop your self-care plan, think about your unique needs and how you can build initiatives into your routine to meet them in positive ways.

Ultimately, when human beings are overworked, overstressed, and not taking care of their needs, they will eventually burn out.[15] We may even hurt what we're trying to protect by failing to take care of ourselves. For instance, my attorney client Ethan spent so many years working on stressful corporate mergers and neglecting his own well-being that he suffered a heart attack. This event inspired him to slow down and add more self-care into his life. Career, family commitments, and social obligations all thrive when we show up for them fully present and healthy.

Individuals practice self-care through many avenues such as building on healthy lifestyle habits, creating routines, and consistently going to preventative medical appointments. Self-care may also be achieved by engaging in activities that enrich life—for instance, travel, hobbies, puzzles, or digging into a new book. I like what Jean Shinoda Bolen said about this: "When you recover or discover something that nourishes your soul and brings joy, care enough about yourself to make room for it in your life." Self-care may even be inaction. Consider taking a pause, allowing the mind and body to rest.

Self-care should be practical. It's not about extremes or all-or-nothing mentality. Consider ways to realistically align self-care with your existing lifestyle. Design an approach that will work for you. Mitch originally wanted to take evening workout classes, but he found he was too tired at the end of the day. When he switched to morning workouts, his weekly routine went more smoothly *and* he felt better at day's end. Emily shifted her cooking-heavy nutrition plan when her professional circumstances required her to travel weekly. George initially experimented with intermittent fasting but needed to tweak his window so he could enjoy meals with his family. Anna found that she needed to plan her vacations far in advance and alert her work team. This lessened her anxiety around taking time off.

Take into consideration your own preferences and motivators. Likes and dislikes matter exponentially. It's tough to follow through on lifestyle initiatives if they are irksome or inconvenient. Keep this in mind when choosing an exercise routine, dietary pattern, mindfulness strategy, or bedtime routine. Past failures also serve as great feedback. We are creatures of habit, so when something consistently doesn't work, it's time to experiment with a new approach. Further, long-term routines that isolate an individual from others may become problematic. Marie discovered this when she was training for the Chicago Marathon. For four months she spent all her free time running, following a strict dietary protocol, and avoiding social gatherings with family and friends. After the race, she concluded that she needed a more balanced approach to staying in shape in the off-season that allowed her more opportunities to fully engage with loved ones. There are many ways to be healthy and reach lifestyle goals. Find the approach that best suits your wheel of harmony.

Finally, give yourself grace. Appreciate that life happens. Life events like an exceptionally busy work period, illness, travel, or holidays may derail regular self-care routines. Don't throw in the towel and allow these instances to stop you from practicing self-care altogether. Recognize it as a normal part of life and focus on moving forward. I wear a gold necklace engraved with the word *grace* as a reminder.

Remember, self-care is not a test or a competition. Self-care should be viewed over time, not in one day, one week, or a few challenging months. The following chapters are about learning what works for you and how to shift to a place of harmonious wellness. It's not about winning. It's more about realizing that *something* is always better than nothing. Stay flexible and modify as necessary to fit current life happenings. Even during the busiest of times, allow yourself pockets of self-care—five minutes of movement, two minutes of breath work, a protein-rich snack, and at least six hours of sleep. You are worth it!

Examples of Self-Care:

Spending Time with
Loved Ones and Pets

Setting & Maintaining
Boundaries

Spending Time
in Nature

Movie or
Game Night

Eating Well

Restorative Sleep

Saying No

Lighting a Candle

Moving Your Body
Consistently

Diffusing
Essential Oil

Massage or
Taking a Bath

Listening to Music
or a Podcast

Meditating

Deep Breathing

Having No Plans

Reading a Book

Haircut or
Manicure

Preventative Doctor &
Dental Appointments

SELF-CARE
ASSESSMENT

Self-care means taking time to do the things that you enjoy and incorporating positive supports into your routine that will increase your mental and physical well-being.

Take a moment to consider how often you are engaging in different self-care practices. The goal is to recognize patterns in your life and consider areas that may require more of your attention. This is meant to be a judgment-free exercise and there are no right or wrong answers.

Consider your self-care frequency on the following scale:

1 – I do this rarely or not at all
2 – I do this sometimes
3 – I do this often

After you have completed the assessment, go back and heart ♥ or star ★ the areas you would like to increase your frequency in to better support your self-care needs.

Physical Self-Care

1   2   3   ♥/★ ————————————————

☐ ☐ ☐   ☐   Eat healthy foods

☐ ☐ ☐   ☐   Take care of my personal hygiene
(i.e., brushing teeth, flossing,
shower, bath)

☐ ☐ ☐   ☐   Exercise

☐ ☐ ☐   ☐   Wear clothes that make me feel
good about myself

☐ ☐ ☐   ☐   Eat homecooked meals

☐ ☐ ☐   ☐   Participate in enjoyable activities
(i.e., walking, group fitness class,
sports, dancing)

☐ ☐ ☐   ☐   Sleep seven to nine hours per night

☐ ☐ ☐   ☐   Go to preventative medical
appointments (i.e., annual exams,
dental cleanings)

☐ ☐ ☐   ☐   Engage in relaxing activities (i.e.,
massage, bath, reading, listening
to music)

☐ ☐ ☐   ☐   Move throughout the day (i.e.,
taking the stairs, getting up from
my desk to stretch)

————————————————————————

Mental / Emotional Self-Care

1	2	3	♥/★	
☐	☐	☐	☐	Use my vacation and PTO time
☐	☐	☐	☐	Engage in hobbies that I enjoy
☐	☐	☐	☐	Disconnect from technology (i.e., technology cutoff time, social media break)
☐	☐	☐	☐	Engage in personal development (i.e., take a class, learn a new skill)
☐	☐	☐	☐	Express my feelings in a healthy way (i.e., therapy, talking to a friend, journaling, creating art, playing music)
☐	☐	☐	☐	Laugh
☐	☐	☐	☐	Spend quality time with family, friends, and pets
☐	☐	☐	☑	Set and maintain personal boundaries
☐	☐	☐	☐	Practice gratitude
☐	☐	☐	☐	Practice self-compassion and positive self-talk

Social Self-Care

1	2	3	♥/★	
☐	☐	☐	☐	Connect with old friends that I do not see regularly (i.e., Zoom, phone call, email)
☐	☐	☐	☐	Engage in enjoyable activities with loved ones, friends, and pets (i.e., game night, potluck dinner, walk in nature)
☐	☐	☐	☐	Spend time alone with my romantic partner or open to connecting with others
☐	☐	☐	☐	Engage in a supportive community (i.e., recovery group, book club, social sports league)
☐	☐	☐	☐	Say yes to social invitations
☐	☐	☐	☐	Celebrate holidays and special occasions with loved ones
☐	☐	☐	☐	Attend community events (i.e., farmer's market, sports game, theater production, festival)
☐	☐	☐	☐	Establish healthy social boundaries and freely use my No button
☐	☐	☐	☐	Engage with like-minded individuals (i.e., online forum, meetup interest group, cooking class)
☐	☐	☐	☐	Work to maintain current relationships and build new ones

Spiritual Self-Care

1	2	3	♥/★	
☐	☐	☐	☐	Practice meditation or prayer
☐	☐	☐	☐	Spend time in nature
☐	☐	☐	☐	Take mindful pauses in my day to shut out the noise (i.e., breath work, repeating a mantra, pausing before acting)
☐	☐	☐	☐	Recognize the things that bring meaning to my life (i.e., gratitude, glass half full)
☐	☐	☐	☐	Live according to my values
☐	☐	☐	☐	Engage in philanthropy and volunteer work
☐	☐	☐	☐	Participate in activities that nurture my spirit and give me purpose
☐	☐	☐	☐	Journal to connect with my deeper self
☐	☐	☐	☐	Connect with a spiritual community (i.e., church, yoga class, recovery group)
☐	☐	☐	☐	Read inspirational books, stories, or listen to a motivational podcast

Professional Self-Care

1	2	3	♥/★	
☐	☐	☐	☐	Engage in continuing education
☐	☐	☐	☐	Set and maintain boundaries regarding my work schedule and nonemergency work emails and calls after hours
☐	☐	☐	☐	Know my daily energy and work-flow to schedule accordingly (i.e., morning person, afternoon slump, energized in the evening)
☐	☐	☐	☐	Recognize my limit when I am taking on too much and ask for assistance
☐	☐	☐	☐	Take on projects or clients that are interesting and rewarding
☐	☐	☐	☐	Maintain harmony between my personal and professional lives
☐	☐	☐	☐	Maintain a mindful and organized workspace
☐	☐	☐	☐	Build and maintain healthy relationships with colleagues
☐	☐	☐	☐	Engage in professional organizations
☐	☐	☐	☐	Take breaks during my workday to recharge (i.e., eat a healthy meal, go for a walk, listen to an energizing song, meditate, breath work)

5 | CREATE FLEXIBLE ROUTINES

What you do every day matters more than what you do once in a while.

—GRETCHEN RUBIN

WHILE I WAS in graduate school studying to be a mental health counselor, my physical and mental well-being suffered greatly. Ironic, I know! With classes, my clinical internship, work, and my family, I overextended myself. One day I woke up with a high fever and couldn't even swallow a glass of water. I was laid up in bed for two weeks, the sickest I had ever been. My body literally forced me to take time off from my crazy life. It was a huge wake-up call for me. Clearly, I was doing too much—school, work, board meetings, wellness presentations, daily morning workouts, social obligations.

Building healthy routines saved me. Where I'd always been an all-or-nothing achiever, I began to practice healthy lifestyle habits in smaller pockets of self-care. These days I share this strategy with all my professional clients because it works. I am a firm believer that no matter your profession or how busy life gets, you have ten minutes a day to devote to self-care. This adds up to seventy minutes a week, which is a perfect place to start. We could all find ten minutes if we made it a priority. Think about how many hours a week we spend browsing online, scrolling social media, dillydallying around the house or office, or stressing about the future, past, or present. Instead, we can put that ten minutes to good use.

As busy individuals, we often feel like we do not have enough time to practice self-care. Exercising, meditating, sleeping, eating lunch, going to the doctor, and using vacation days takes time. Neglecting to invest in self-care, however, creates chronic stress, preventable diseases, and mental health concerns.[16] Professionals grappling with substance misuse and addiction often believe they have no time for treatment. Tim initially felt like this but realized that if he wanted to maintain his career, relationships, and health he needed to make space for his recovery.

Some people find it challenging to reorganize their lives to support self-care needs. Routines provide structure and manageability. They promote physical, mental, and emotional well-being. The absence of a routine causes tension, burnout, and overwhelm.[17] Routines allow individuals to seamlessly weave healthy lifestyle habits into daily life until they become second nature. Routines also create ease, empowering individuals to maintain their wellness during busy professional and personal seasons.

Bill, a trial lawyer, litigates cases that last for weeks or even months. During these periods, he alters his routines to support his current circumstances. It's precisely during these high-stress periods that Bill needs to weave in self-care to give himself some room to breathe. So he modifies his hour-long workouts to fifteen-to-twenty-minute sessions and gets healthy meals delivered to his office. Gia's schedule changes each summer when her children are off from school. She reads a novel while her kids are at swim practice and cooks healthy meals together as a fun family activity. Logan, who is in medical sales, travels monthly. He utilizes his routine as a base to pivot from when he is on the road to during his weeks at home. When we have routines in place, we can easily resume them when schedules return to a more manageable pace.

Build routines on existing lifestyle habits to support self-care needs. Habits encourage consistency in new behaviors and may also be used to replace unwanted behaviors. Michelle, who works a high-stress job, began taking yoga classes in the evenings instead of ordering fast-food carryout. Start small and build new habits into routines over time. For example, add in five servings of produce per day, track daily steps, meditate for five minutes, and sleep for seven hours.

Updating your environment in small ways encourages new habits and discourages unwanted behaviors. For example, you could discard junk food from the pantry and desk, remove storage items off the treadmill to make it easier to access, delete a social media app, or download a meditation app. Additionally, some individuals find success by "stacking" new habits around activities or consistent habits. You always eat dinner, so add an after-dinner walk. After brushing your teeth, write in a gratitude journal. Further, you can break habits down by time increments and amounts. For example, you could start with a ten-minute walk, then increase to twenty minutes, then to thirty minutes. Or begin with cooking a homemade meal two times a week, and then increase to three times and then four times. Furthermore, you can write out a step-by-step plan to develop your habit (i.e., go to bed by ten o'clock every night: brush teeth and wash up by 9:30 p.m., get into bed, read a chapter of a book, and turn off the nightstand light). Moreover, routines allow for a base to stay grounded in wellness whether you work remotely, hybrid, or in an office.

Here is a go-to formula for developing morning, evening, and workday routines. Read through the structure below and begin by crafting at least one daily routine, and then develop the others over time. Building routines and healthy habits will be an essential component of your future SMART goal setting in part 3 of this book.

A.M. ROUTINE

- Rise at a consistent time. Skip the snooze button.

- Engage in something positive to set an optimistic mood for the day, such as:

  - ★ Exercise.

  - ★ Practice mindfulness—
    meditate, gratitude journal, no phone.

  - ★ Walk the dog or take care
    of any household pets.

  - ★ If you have children, get them
    ready for the day.

- ★ Read the newspaper or your preferred news feed with a coffee or tea.

- ★ Eat a nutritious breakfast with protein.

- Complete your dental and skin-care routine.

- Shower and dress in a professional, smart casual, or athleisure attire—people are much more motivated for work and life out of pj's.

WORKDAY ROUTINE

- Eat healthy meals and snacks, even when working remotely.

  - ★ Grocery shop, meal prep, and pack meals and snacks for the week.

    - ♥ Keep it simple: repeat meals, use bento boxes, repurpose leftovers.

  - ★ Print out carryout menus and highlight go-to meals and snacks.

- Make movement a part of the day.

  - ★ Go for a ten-minute walk.

- ★ Take stretch breaks or do desk exercises like shoulder rolls, arm circles, alternating knee lifts, or stand up and do side bends.

- Engage in a mindfulness break.

  - ★ Spend five minutes on meditation or breath work.

  - ★ Practice gratitude by writing down or thinking on five things that you are grateful for each day.

- Create a supportive environment to set a positive tone in your workspace by keeping it tidy and including plants, a water bottle, photos, artwork, or a favorite screen saver.

P.M. ROUTINE

After-work wind-down:

- Change clothes as a mental and physical cue to transition from the workday—even for remote workers.

- Eat a nutritious meal.

- ★ This would be a great time to pack meals and snacks for the next day.

- Spend time with loved ones.

- Decompress by going for a walk, watching a TV show, or playing board games.

- Lay out clothes for the next morning.

  - ★ On Sunday, choose five outfits for the whole workweek.

ACTION ITEM: BUILD DAILY ROUTINES

A.M. Routine

What is your consistent rise time? _____

What habits will you engage in to prep for a positive mindset and daily outcome?

Habit 1: _____

Habit 2: _____

Habit 3: _____

P.M. Routine

How will you transition from work mode? _____

_____

_____

What habits will you engage in to wind down from your busy day?

Habit 1: _____

Habit 2: _____

Habit 3: _____

Workday Routine

What will you do to create a supportive work environment?

_____

_____

_____

_____

_____

What habits will you engage in to promote self-care and create a successful workday?

Habit 1: _____

Habit 2: _____

Habit 3: _____

6 | FITNESS FOR THE BUSY PROFESSIONAL

*If exercise could be packaged in a pill,
it would be the single most widely
prescribed and beneficial medicine
in the nation.*

—Robert Butler
National Institute on Aging

I've competed in more than my fair share of cheer and dance competitions. Our pom squad excelled in the kick competition, and we used to perform numbers like the Radio City Rockettes. My favorite was a routine to the eighties hit "Gloria." I even coached my high school pom squad when I was in college. I pushed my developing body past its physical limits on a regular basis, and then I carried my extreme mindset around fitness into adulthood. Looking back, I see how obsessive I was. Between daily strength training sessions, Pilates classes, and cardio, I never took a day off. It took a physical toll on my body and soon it began to negatively impact my mental health. When my knees and emotional health finally broke down, I knew it was time for a change. I needed to embrace a new fitness mentality. Now I train less intensely and focus on exercises that support my body instead of harming it. I enjoy fitness again! I give myself rest days and strengthen my recovery with physical therapy and other holistic practices such as massage, needling, and hot/cold therapy.

Professionals often grapple with making time in their busy schedules for regular physical activity. Some individuals may also feel discouraged about their current level of fitness. For example, Janice had not exercised in years and admitted she felt embarrassed about going to the gym. Mark played baseball in college when life afforded him time to train for hours. He wanted to play on a community softball team but was frustrated with his fitness level, so he kept putting it off. Harper used to enjoy hour-long spin classes several times a week. Now she felt like her career and parenting responsibilities afforded her little time for exercise.

Wellness practitioners support a thoughtful and balanced approach to fitness.[18] For Janice, that meant working out in a more private setting, like a home gym. For Mark, joining the recreational team allowed him to play at a much less intense level and enjoy it more. For Harper, it meant completing shorter workouts throughout the week, including neighborhood walks and bike rides with her family. In all three cases, small changes made a big difference.

According to researchers, exercise is the number one lifestyle strategy to increase lifespan and longevity. It prevents and lowers an individual's risk for diseases such as heart disease, cancer, and dementia.[19] Exercise also supports weight loss or weight maintenance. Staying active physically helps maintain muscle mass and bone density, and it guards against a condition called sarcopenia, the loss of skeletal muscle mass and strength as we age.[20]

Beyond the physical benefits, exercise greatly improves overall mental health and neurological functioning.[21] As Elle Woods cleverly noted in *Legally Blonde*, "Exercise gives you endorphins. Endorphins make you happy." Simply moving regularly boosts mood, improves one's ability to cope with daily stressors, and mitigates disorders like depression and anxiety.

Physical activity guidelines for adults define "moderate exercise" as working out approximately one hundred and fifty minutes a week at an intensity that a person can get their heart rate up to 70 to 85 percent of their predicted maximum heart rate (the number 220 minus your age), or the intensity of a brisk walk.[22] This means it's only 1.5 percent of your week, or roughly twenty minutes a day! Experts also encourage at least two days of strength training per week. This makes a lot of practical sense.

Years ago, I was at a wellness talk at Canyon Ranch in Lenox, Massachusetts. The exercise physiologist noted that cardio gives years to your life and strength training gives life to your years. In other words, a healthy heart may extend an individuals' life, but strong bones and muscles allow them to perform activities of daily living like carrying groceries, climbing the stairs, and getting into and out of a car. I also advise my female clients, who might be more accustomed to cardio, to add strength training to their weekly fitness routines. This is especially important when women transition through menopause, which is associated with a loss of bone mass density, muscle mass, and strength.[23] It can further assist with hormonal weight gain.

I encourage clients to focus their exercise routines to support their wheel of harmony. It's normal for fitness to shift over time due to life circumstances, age, injuries, new goals, and even boredom. For example, Pam exercises at her local gym for thirty minutes five days a week, doing a combination of cardio and strength training. Janey walks her dog every day and completes two weekly strength training workouts online. Max takes a HIIT class three days a week over his lunch hour. My husband, John, is a weekend warrior and completes two longer workouts on Saturday and Sunday. Jeanne prefers to garden, swim laps, and play with her grandchildren. Morgan gets some of her exercise in by walking fifteen minutes to and from the train station. Kris plays in an adult hockey league with his college buddies. Grace bought her family members activity trackers for Christmas, and they motivate each other. My point is that there are many ways to fit movement into a busy life.

In this current age of technology, many individuals sit at desks all day or look down on smartphones. Traditional advice to take the stairs or park at the end of the lot all enhance daily movement. Strive to get in three scheduled workouts a week and be active in life. Here are a few healthy habits and strategies to build a consistent exercise routine:

- Start by scheduling set workouts in your calendar and treat them like any other appointment. Move them to another day or time if something *important* comes up. Consider exercising a boundary you are setting with yourself.

- If you feel tired or pressed for time, shorten your workout to stay consistent.

- Exercise during workdays. Go for a walk or to the gym/studio over the lunch hour. Walk or bike to and from work or the train station. Strength train in a private or home office with exercise bands, desk exercises, or bodyweight exercises.

- Set movement alarms every hour or two during the workday on a smartphone or watch. When the alarm goes off, get up for a few minutes to stretch or walk around the office/home.

- Invest in a fitness tracker, such as a Fitbit, Apple Watch, or WHOOP, to record daily steps and movement. You can set a daily steps goal (i.e., 5,000–10,000 steps per day) and increase it over time.

- Set workout clothes and gym shoes out the night before (or pack them to go) as a helpful reminder of tomorrow's planned workout.

- Find a buddy or colleague to help you stay motivated and accountable. Office challenges are also a great way to build camaraderie and get work teams moving together.

- Exercise with your family. Go for a walk after dinner to connect and get steps in. Take a workout class or create a family challenge through an activity tracker or app.

- Join a community sports league to enhance your social supports.

- Make recovery a part of your routine with rest days and holistic practices like massage, acupuncture, and hot/cold therapy (steam, sauna, Epsom salt baths, cold plunge/shower). These practices are also great for relaxation and stress management.

- Stop making excuses!

Now take a moment to map out a consistent exercise routine. Start by selecting three days a week for planned exercise and note three healthy habits or strategies to set you up for success. Start small if necessary. Even walking for fifteen minutes three days a week is a great place to begin and grow. Think about how your exercise routine can align and enhance your wheel of harmony.

ACTION ITEM: EXERCISE ROUTINE

Exercise Routine

What days and times are doable for three workouts per week?

_____

_____

_____

What habits will set you up for success?

Habit 1: _____

Habit 2: _____

Habit 3: _____

What will you do to support your recovery (i.e., stretching, massage, sauna, steam, Epsom salt bath, foam rolling)?

_____

_____

7 | EAT WELL

One cannot think well,
love well, or sleep well,
if one has not dined well.

—Virginia Woolf

THE TOPIC OF nutrition is ripe with contradictions. Just look online and a new diet trend is emerging as the hot new way to be fit and healthy. Many of these plans are gimmicky and expensive, not to mention restrictive and challenging to maintain. My intention in these pages is to help you view nutrition through a holistic lens.

The nutrition chapter has been by far the most challenging for me to write. I wrestled with food and eating disorders for many years. I pursued training and education around it as well. So I have strong feelings about food, ample knowledge about nutrition, and a depth of experience working with food-related issues. My philosophy about food can be summarized with one word: harmony.

My background as a health coach and mental health counselor gives me special empathy for those who have struggled with food. From experience I can attest that it can be enormously painful and will take time to heal both behaviorally and emotionally. My approach will always be one of support and encouragement.

Healthy nutrition is not just about physical needs and a number on the scale. Mental and emotional well-being play a key role. While human beings need food to *physically* survive, *emotional* health is impacted too. For example, food can be celebratory; bring comfort, joy, shame, or sadness; and offer escape. Nutrition ideally allows individuals to thrive in their wheel of harmony by maximizing energy and overall wellness.

While there are many approaches to nutrition, most health professionals agree that individuals need to shift their dietary pattern away from the Standard American Diet. SAD has been known to play a key role in the obesity epidemic and is associated with chronic diseases like diabetes, cardiovascular disease, and some cancers.[24] Americans eat high amounts of ultra-processed foods—soft drinks, fried foods, sweetened breakfast cereals—and fewer nutritious foods like fruits and vegetables.[25] Beyond physical concerns, SAD is associated with a higher risk of depression, anxiety, and mental health disorders.[26]

A simple way for individuals to dial up their nutrition is by leaning into a more nutrient-dense dietary pattern comprising whole foods—vegetables, fruits, meat, poultry, fish, nuts, seeds, whole grains, beans, legumes, and healthy fats. Unlike SAD, this way of eating has been associated with reduced risk of chronic disease and decreased instances of mental health disorders.[27] It also increases the overall quality of life across the wheel of harmony. For instance, my husband, John, is a first-generation American, and his family comes together as a community to share foods from the Mediterranean tradition of Greece. He not only is enjoying delicious healthy foods but also is supporting his emotional wellness by sharing laughs with loved ones and connecting to his roots.

Beyond basic nutritional principles, there are numerous dietary patterns for people to choose from—balanced, low-carb, high-protein, vegan, paleo, intermittent fasting, and intuitive eating. Barring any specific medical diagnosis or food sensitivities, individuals have the most success when they eat according to their personal preferences. Regardless of which dietary plan a person chooses, it's the ability to stick to the plan that predicts long-term success. In other words, people should choose a way of eating that is nourishing and doable on a consistent basis.[28]

Busy people often find success when they follow a specific nutrition strategy. A plan helps professionals navigate common nutrition mishaps like skipping meals, stress eating, yo-yo dieting, and overcomplication. Like a routine, dietary patterns provide a base to work from and return to when life interrupts the routine (vacation, busy work period, personal crisis). Dietary patterns typically follow one of three strategies:

Calorie Restriction: balanced approach. This is the old-school method of counting calories or macronutrients. This way of eating is the most flexible dietary pattern and allows people to enjoy their favorite foods in moderation. Initially, it does require individuals to record daily food and drink consumption as well as measure or eyeball food servings. My grandma, who had a sweet tooth, ate with a balanced approach so she was able to enjoy her traditional Polish foods.

Macro or Dietary Restriction: low-fat, low-carb, vegetarian, vegan, keto, paleo. This method excludes an entire food group—no animal products, sugar, carbs, or fat. Some individuals find this method easy because they just avoid or limit certain foods. Others find it challenging in the long run. For instance, Dina rebounded into yo-yo dieting when she completely restricted her carb intake.

Time Restriction: intermittent fasting. This method works well for individuals who prefer to eat all their food in a time-restricted window. The 16:8 method, where you consume all your food in an eight-hour window, is very popular. For example, an individual may consume food only from 12 p.m. to 8 p.m. or from 8 a.m. to 4 p.m. This approach can occasionally be challenging depending on work and family schedules. For example, David needed to shift his fasting window to have dinner with his children. Also, individuals need to still consume an adequate amount of protein and other nutrients.

Choose the dietary pattern that works best for your wheel of harmony. You can then use the following Erin Clifford Wellness (ECW) plates and healthy habits to put it into practice. Make it part of your routine.

ECW PLATES

ECW Balanced Plate

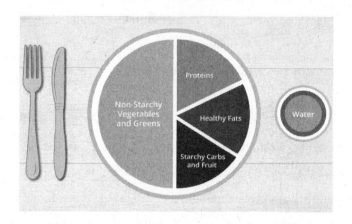

ECW Low-Fat Plate

Dial up the carbs and dial down the fat.

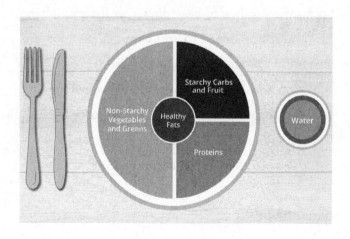

ECW Low-Carb Plate

Dial down the carbs and dial up the fat.

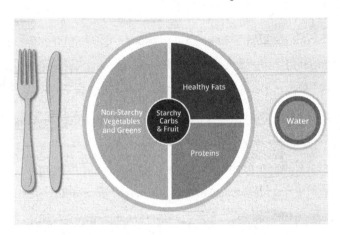

ECW Time-Restricted Eating

Limit eating to eight to twelve waking hours each day.

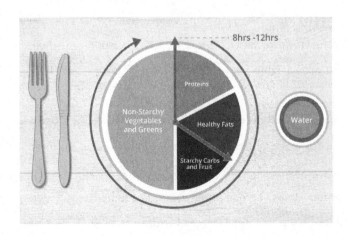

Assemble your preferred ECW plate with the following macronutrients:

Protein: Build your plate around protein-rich foods spread throughout the day. A serving is generally 4 oz. for women and 6 oz. for men.

Non-Starchy Vegetables and Greens: Enjoy 1–2 servings per meal to boost health and daily fiber intake. For example, enjoy a side salad, oven-roasted vegetables, or sautéed green beans with your meal. You can also eat baby carrots, cucumbers, and bell pepper slices with hummus for a snack, or celery sticks with peanut butter. A serving size is 1/2 cup cooked or 1 cup raw vegetables and 2 cups raw greens.

Healthy Fats: Based on your chosen dietary pattern, dial your fat up or down. A serving is 1 tablespoon olive oil, 10 nuts, 1 tablespoon seeds, or 1/3 avocado.

Starchy Carbohydrates and Fruit: Based on your chosen dietary pattern, dial your starchy carbohydrates and fruit up or down. A serving is 1 slice Ezekiel bread, 1/2 cup whole grains, 1 small sweet potato, 1 cup berries, 1/2 cup sliced fruit, or 1 small piece of fruit.

PROTEIN

Protein is essential for building and repairing muscle, regulating hormones, and supporting an individual's immune system. Protein also helps with weight maintenance and curbing cravings throughout the day. As a rule of thumb, build meals and snacks around the protein component.

Active and older adults require additional protein. Research recommends consuming at least 1.6 grams per kilogram of body weight per day (or approximately .7 grams per pound) as the minimum and up to 2.2 grams per kilogram of body weight per day (or approximately 1 gram per pound) for active individuals with normal kidney function.[29] For example, Bill, who weighs 68 kilograms, or 150 pounds, needs 108.8–150 grams of protein per day (weight in kilograms and multiply by 1.6–2.2) depending on his lifestyle goals. Consult with a doctor or nutritionist about specific protein needs.

Recommended serving sizes of protein:

- 4 oz. serving for women, 6 oz. serving for men—chicken, turkey, lean beef, bison, pork, fish

- 2 eggs or 1/2 cup egg whites

- Protein powder (vegan, bone broth, or collagen from grass-fed cows)

- 4 oz. tofu

- 1/2 cup lentils or beans

- 3/4 cup chickpea pasta, lentil pasta

- 1/4 cup hummus

- 1 oz. cheese

- 1/2 cup cottage cheese

- 1 cup unsweetened Greek yogurt, coconut yogurt, almond yogurt, or cashew yogurt

- 1 cup milk, unsweetened almond milk, coconut milk, or hemp seed milk

VEGETABLES AND FRUIT

Eating the colors of the rainbow is crucial for optimal nutrition. Fruits and vegetables provide human beings with vitamins, minerals, and dietary fiber, and they lower the risk of chronic diseases like heart disease, obesity, and some cancers.[30] Leafy greens like kale also reduce depression and improve mood.[31]

Leafy Greens (2 cup servings—if this feels like a lot of greens you can cook it down like sautéed spinach or add it to a soup or smoothie)

> arugula, chicory, collard, endive, escarole, iceberg lettuce, kale, mustard, radicchio, romaine, spinach, turnip, watercress

Non-starchy Vegetables (1/2 cup servings)

> artichoke, asparagus, bamboo shoots, bean sprouts, beets, broccoli, brussels sprouts, cabbage (green, Bok choy, Chinese), carrots (raw), cauliflower, celery, cucumber, daikon, eggplant, fennel, fermented vegetables, leeks, greens, mushrooms, okra, onions, pea pods, peppers, radishes, rutabaga, squash, sugar snap peas, Swiss chard, tomato, water chestnuts, zucchini (zoodles)

Fruit (1/2 large fruit, 1 medium-sized fruit, 1 cup berries)

> apples, bananas, blackberries, blueberries, cantaloupe, cherries, mango, nectarines, peaches, pears, pineapple, plums, watermelon

STARCHY CARBS

So-called slow carbohydrates like starchy vegetables and whole grains are absorbed more slowly than other carbs and do not cause a rapid spike in insulin. Slow carbs can also help crush cravings and increase fiber and nutrients.[32]

Starchy Vegetables (1/2 cup servings)

> beets, carrots (cooked), corn on the cob, parsnips, potatoes (new, red, russet, sweet), pumpkin, squash (acorn, butternut, spaghetti), yam

Whole Grains, Breads, and Pasta (1/2 cup serving whole grains or cereal, 3/4 cup pasta, 1 slice bread, 1/2 bagel or 1/2 English muffin)

> amaranth, barley, bread (Ezekiel sprouted grain, sourdough, whole grain), buckwheat, cassava tortilla (2 small), corn tortilla (2 small), couscous (whole grain), millet, pasta (brown rice, whole grain, lentil, bean), pita bread (1/2 6-inch whole grain), quinoa, rice (black, brown, wild), steel cut oats, tortilla (6-inch sprouted grain, whole grain, or brown rice), whole grain cereal (unsweetened)

HEALTHY FATS

Healthy fats are pivotal to achieving optimal wellness and brain health. Monounsaturated fats (olive oil, avocados, nuts) and polyunsaturated fats (Omega-6 and Omega-3) have a positive effect on health when eaten in moderation. Omega-3 fats are extremely beneficial in reducing symptoms of depression and anxiety, and they help prevent chronic conditions like cardiovascular disease, diabetes, some cancers, and dementia.[33]

When cooking with fats, be aware of the smoke points of oils. Grapeseed oil, avocado oil, coconut oil, butter, and ghee (clarified butter) all have high smoke points. Olive oil does not. Refrain from grilling with olive oil. Instead, use it to make a salad dressing or drizzle on vegetables.

Further, limit cooking and consuming foods containing canola oil, sunflower seed oil, corn oil, and soybean oil. These oils are commonly used to prolong the shelf-life of ultra-processed foods. Studies now suggest that consuming a high quantity of these oils may increase inflammation in the body and contribute to disease.[34]

Oils (1 tablespoon)
avocado oil, coconut oil, extra-virgin olive oil, ghee, grass-fed butter, MCT oil, walnut oil

Nuts and Seeds

almonds (12), Brazil nuts (3–4), cashews (9), hazelnuts (10), macadamia nuts (5–6), pecans (10 halves), peanuts (20), pistachios (20–22), walnuts (7 halves); 1 tablespoon: chia seeds, flaxseeds, hemp seeds, poppy seeds, pumpkin seeds, sesame seeds, sunflower seeds; 1 tablespoon: unsweetened nut butters or tahini

Additional Fats

1 tablespoon: avocado mayonnaise, pesto, sour cream; 10 small black or large green olives; 4 large black or kalamata olives; 1/3 avocado

WATER

Hydration is key. The National Academies of Sciences, Engineering, and Medicine recommends adult males need approximately 15.5 cups (3.7 liters) of fluids per day, and adult women need approximately 11.5 cups (2.7 liters) of fluids per day.[35]

Avoid sugary beverages such as soda, vitamin water, artificially flavored sparkling water, and sports drinks. Instead, flavor water with your favorite fruits. You can do this easily by using a water bottle or pitcher with a fruit infuser.

HEALTHY HABITS TO OPTIMIZE YOUR DIETARY STRATEGY

Follow the 80/20 Approach

Eighty percent of the time, make mindful, nutrient-dense food choices that are going to be beneficial to the body and mind. The other 20 percent of the time include favorite comfort foods, indulgences, and traditional foods. Unless an individual has a food sensitivity, no food should be off-limits. The key is to practice overall balance and moderation.

Crowd in the Rainbow

Instead of thinking about what you *can't* have, crowd in nutrients by eating at least five servings of colorful fruits and vegetables each day. As a rule of thumb, fill half the plate with vegetables and greens at lunch and dinner.

Up Fiber Intake

Fiber is extremely important for regulating gastrointestinal (GI) health, cholesterol, and preventing disease. It also increases satiety, so people are less likely to fill up on empty calories.

According to the Mayo Clinic, women should eat at least 21 to 25 grams of fiber a day, while men should aim for 30 to 38 grams a day. Foods with a higher fiber content are vegetables, fruits, legumes, nuts, seeds, and whole grains. Individuals may also consult with their doctors about fiber supplements.

Smart Snacking

While it might be tempting to snack to alleviate stress and boredom, choose healthier options to boost energy and satiety. Include a protein and fiber component—hummus and vegetables, almond butter and an apple, smoothie, yogurt and berries, or string cheese and whole grain crackers.

Drink Alcohol in Moderation

Be mindful of alcohol intake. Alcohol contains a lot of empty calories, and it can have a negative impact on immunity, hormones, and sleep.[36] Alcohol further increases an individual's risk for chronic disease and cancer. It's also an appetite inducer and causes people to make unhealthy food choices. I remind my clients to be mindful of the next day "crave over."

Choose hard alcohol alone or mixed with seltzer (such as a vodka soda, tequila with pineapple) or a glass of wine. Stay away from sugary mixed drinks, such as a frozen margarita or daiquiri. Individuals who are reducing carbs should be mindful of beers and ciders.

Monitor Caffeine Intake

Be sure to monitor your caffeine intake. Generally, most individuals need to cut off caffeine by 2 p.m. or it may affect their sleep.[37] Also, if you struggle with anxiety, limit your caffeine consumption.

Track Food, Drink, and Fiber Intake

Keeping track of food and beverage intake is a smart way to stay accountable and track progress. Use a digital app like MyFitnessPal or write in a food journal. When tracking calories and macros digitally, use the same entry each time for a specific food. For example, always use the same grilled chicken entry. While calorie/macro tracking is not an accurate science, being consistent will help gauge progress.

If this seems overwhelming, just track protein and fiber intake. In addition, tracking will help identify any behaviors that are inhibiting you from reaching wellness goals. For instance, Sherry observed that she was consuming some of her child's leftovers in addition to her own meals. Todd recognized that every time he passed his assistant's candy dish, he grabbed a few pieces.

Be a Conscious Consumer

Read food labels carefully when selecting foods at the grocery or in takeaway food shops. Check out the nutrition facts panel and the ingredients list. The more ingredients, the more processed a food. As a rule of thumb, if you do not know what an ingredient is, you do not want to put it in your body.

The Kitchen Is Closed After Dinner

Go at least twelve hours between dinner and breakfast. This is called a "circadian rhythm fast" and is a shorter form of time-restricted eating. This allows the GI system to rest and, from a behavioral standpoint, discourages late-night snacking, which is when people are more prone to eat empty calories (ice cream, candy, chips).

Practice Mindful Eating

- Eat without distractions such as television and social media.

- Eat at the kitchen table or counter when possible. Avoid eating in the workspace.

- Put the fork down between bites, and take a sip of water or engage in conversation.

- Eat until you are 80 percent full.

- Ask yourself if you are hungry or simply stressed, bored, excited, and so on. If you are not sure, drink a glass of water first. You may be dehydrated.

Eat at Set Mealtimes

Many workaholics often forget to eat and then are ravenous by the end of the day. They then overeat one huge meal and often turn to fast food or high-calorie options for convenience. To avoid this, eat at consistent mealtimes and set an alarm as a reminder to not skip meals.

Cook and Meal Prep

One of the best forms of self-care is cooking homemade meals and consistently bringing meals and snacks to work. As a bonus, it's much more cost effective. See appendix A for a meal planning guide. Overall, your nutrition strategy should not be complicated. Simply choose a dietary pattern that works for your wheel of harmony. You can then build healthy habits over time to make nutrition an integral part of your self-care routine.

8 | MINDFUL STRESS MANAGEMENT

You can't stop the waves,
but you can learn how to surf.

—Jon Kabat-Zinn

STRESS HAS A branding problem. All human beings experience stress, which can be positive or negative. Beneficial stress (aka "eustress") motivates and helps individuals thrive in challenging situations. I often feel *eustress* before facilitating a corporate wellness presentation. I experience it as a sort of excitement. On the flip side, *distress* is demotivating and unpleasant. It reminds me of not wanting to get out of bed in the morning when I've suffered a loss. This detrimental form of stress undermines health and functioning across all life domains. Distress is what people are lamenting about when they say they are overly stressed.

When individuals are chronically stressed, their whole wheel of harmony is impacted. It leads to diminished productivity, poor decision-making, reduced creativity, and increased risk of burnout.[38] For example, Barry experienced physical symptoms when he struggled to keep up with the demands at his workplace. Sally grappled with her own mental health concerns when her son began having difficulties in school. We all experience ups and downs from time to time, whether they come as family struggles, relationship problems, health concerns, workplace and financial concerns, or environmental stressors. While it's unrealistic to eliminate stress completely, we can mindfully manage it by building resilience.

Resilience is the capacity to rebound from adversity, trauma, or stress by adapting effectively. When you have resilience, you're like a superhero in disguise.[39] You've got a secret weapon that allows you to thrive despite challenging circumstances. Resilient thoughts and behaviors can be learned and developed in anyone. A great way to enhance resilience is through mindful stress management.

Mindfulness, or the "science of chill," can yield big benefits when it comes to navigating a busy life. Mindfulness involves deliberate slowing of the parasympathetic nervous system through intention.[40] While there are many ways to practice mindfulness, the main tenet is slowing down to be present in the moment without judgment, and refraining from thinking about the past or stressing about the future. Studies show that mindfulness interventions improve physical and mental health, reducing depression, anxiety, perceived stress, and ruminative thinking.[41] Mindfulness practices encourage rest and provide emotional grounding, ultimately helping create more fulfillment in the wheel of harmony.

Individuals need to engage in mindfulness practices consistently to reap the full benefits. Regular practice allows individuals to tap into this soothing response when they experience high-stress situations. For instance, by the consistent practice of breath work, Samantha found she was able to easily access a calming response in her nervous system during a particularly combative work meeting.

It's also important to recognize that while control of a situation isn't always possible, control of one's responses is always an option. For example, if Marcie misplaces her car keys, she can either throw a fit or quietly consider where she might have left them. (I wish I had learned this strategy as a child before I spilled ketchup all over my Pink Ladies jacket!) When mindfulness is utilized as a tool, it allows us to ground ourselves in the moment and learn to navigate stressful occurrences more successfully.

It's normal for the concept of mindfulness to seem uncomfortable at first. When I was teaching a stress management class to a group of lawyers, Philip immediately communicated that he was not doing any kind of "woo-woo stuff." The good news is there are many ways to practice mindfulness. As we explore diverse avenues to mindfully manage stress, keep an open mind. Consider one method that will be helpful to adopt into your regular routine.

MEDITATION AND BREATH WORK

A consistent meditation practice or breath work calms the mind, regulates blood pressure, supports the immune system, and enhances brain health. Creating a ritual around meditation can help you develop a consistent practice. Designate a specific time of day and place in the home or office environment. You might enjoy doing guided meditation through apps on your smartphone.

The following meditation is an integral part of my morning routine. It allows me to nonjudgmentally gauge my emotional state so I can better make decisions and engage with others. It provides an opportunity for gratitude and sets a positive intention for the day. This intention may be very specific, or it could be a state of being (calm, grounded, grateful). If you find it challenging to get in touch with your feelings, start by identifying if you are in a positive, neutral, or negative state.

Daily Mindfulness Check-In

Step 1: Begin with three deep breaths.

Step 2: Ask yourself:

- How am I feeling physically, mentally, and emotionally?

- What are five things that I am grateful for?

- What is my intention for the day?

Step 3: End with three deep breaths.

There are also many breathing exercises with different counts to engage in. A few favorites are:

Calming Breath

This exercise helps calm your nervous system and is a great way to manage stress.

Step 1: Choose a comfortable seat with your back straight and your body relaxed.

Step 2: Empty the air from your lungs.

Step 3: Breathe in quietly through your nose for two seconds.

Step 4: Hold your breath for three seconds.

Step 5: Exhale for four seconds, pursing your lips like you are blowing out a candle.

Repeat the cycle at least four times. Notice how your mind and body feel.

Counting Breath

This breathing exercise is reminiscent of counting sheep. It is a great way to fall asleep or get back to sleep if you wake up during the night.

Step 1: Comfortably lie down on your back in bed and dim the lights.

Step 2: Breathe in and out to the count of 1. Breathe in and out for 2. Continue counting, breathing in and out all the way up to 10.

Step 3: Once you get to 10, begin counting

down, breathing in and out to 9, and so on
until you get down to 1.

Repeat the cycle as needed.

Humming Bee Breath

This yoga breathing practice can help you relieve stress and
exhale from your body unwanted emotions like anxiety,
irritability, and anger.

Step 1: Choose a comfortable seated position
and close your eyes.

Step 2: Gently place your hands over your ears.

Step 3: Inhale and then exhale, keeping
your mouth closed while you make a loud
humming sound.

Repeat the cycle at least four times.

Pinwheel 4-7-8 Breathing Exercise

This fun rhythmic breathing exercise uses a pinwheel but
can certainly be done without one.

Step 1: Sit with your back straight and your
body relaxed.

Step 2: Empty the air from your lungs.

Step 3: Breathe in quietly through your nose for four seconds.

Step 4: Hold your breath for seven seconds.

Step 5: Exhale, pursing your lips and blowing on the pinwheel for eight seconds.

Repeat the cycle up to four times. Notice how your mind and body feel.

GROUNDING PRACTICES

You may further build resilience and engage in mindfulness by utilizing grounding practices. Smells, soothing music, touching something cold, or tugging on a necklace or bracelet may all emotionally and physically ground you in the moment. For example, when Dina gets anxious at work, she smells a bottle of lavender essential oil that she keeps in her desk drawer. Grounding practices may also be supportive for individuals who suffer from past traumas or PTSD.[42] I often recommend grounding practices to my clients if they need a moment to delay a reaction in a stressful professional or personal situation. The following two exercises can be both very grounding and meditative.

5-4-3-2-1 Technique

- Take in the details of your surroundings using each of your five senses.

- What are five things you can see? Look for small details such as a pattern on the ceiling or an object you never noticed.

- What are four things you can feel? Notice the sensation of clothing on your body or the feeling of the chair you are sitting in.

- What are three things you can hear? Pay special attention to the sounds your mind has tuned out, like a ticking clock or distant traffic.

- What are two things you can smell? Try to notice smells in your environment, like an air freshener or flowers.

- What is one thing you can taste? Carry gum, candy, or small snacks for this step. Pop one in your mouth and focus your attention on the flavors.

Categories

Choose a category and name as many items as you can—movies, books, cereals, sports teams, action heroes, states, countries, animals, colors, cities, fruits and vegetables, and so on.

JOURNALING

Regular journaling allows you to connect with your values, emotions, and personal and professional goals. This practice also provides mental clarity and creates more focus across the wheel of harmony. Journals also serve as artifacts of personal history that are enjoyable to read over time.

PRAYER AND RELIGIOUS SERVICES

Prayer is another form of contemplative meditation for those who practice a formal religion. Attending services can also help one feel connected to the larger community.

GRATITUDE

Positive thinking has a tremendous impact on overall wellness.[43] It also helps develop the attitude domain in the wheel of harmony.

Gratitude Journal

Every morning or before you go to bed, write down five things you are grateful for in your life. Revisit your journal any time you need a mental or emotional boost. Some individuals prefer to create a gratitude jar and write things they're grateful for on slips of paper.

Gratitude Walk

If you are a more active person, take a gratitude walk and pay attention to all the beautiful things the natural world has to offer—and get your steps in too. Or go on a gratitude scavenger hunt by looking for something specific on your walk—for instance, dogs, the color blue, pumpkins in the fall, flowers in the spring, and so on.

Gratitude Trigger

Place an object somewhere in your home or workspace that will remind you to feel grateful when you see it. It can be a little sign with your favorite quote, a picture of a loved one, or a screen saver. I have my golden girl, Daisy, as my screen saver.

HOME AND WORK ENVIRONMENT

Create a space that is clutter-free and brings a sense of calm and happiness. Consider deliberate use of joyful objects such as:

- Plants
- Candles
- Essential oils
- Pictures
- Painting or memento

BUILD CONNECTIONS AND SOCIAL SUPPORTS

Connections with others can help reduce stress and anxiety and enhance overall quality of life. Such connections can come from interaction with friends, family, colleagues, or communities.

- Make time for important relationships with family and friends.

- Build new relationships with individuals you connect with.

- Engage in team-building activities with colleagues.

- Increase your community involvement in organizations, clubs, meet-up groups, and sports leagues.

- Use professional supports and join support groups—counselors, coaches, trainers, recovery community.

IDENTIFY AND PLAN FOR HIGH-RISK SITUATIONS

Understanding the effect certain situations and emotions have on you can help you manage these occurrences in a more positive way to reduce your overall stress load. Consider what your high-risk situations are at work (i.e., meeting with superiors, project deadlines, difficult clients) and in your personal life (i.e., holidays, family/in-laws, busy social calendar). When we become more mindful of these challenging situations, we are better able to navigate them and develop a plan for management.

For instance, communicate before and after a high-risk situation to your social supports. Ryan regularly informs his wife when he has a stressful meeting at work and checks in with her afterward. Also, give yourself a way out. When Autumn attends obligatory after-work events, she makes an appearance and has a planned reason to leave early (i.e., early-morning meeting, picking up daughter from soccer practice). Further, schedule intentional self-care. On Christmas, Theo plans a holiday movie night with his children after he leaves his family festivities that are often emotionally dysregulating for him. Additionally, use your self-care avenues and support network to book-mark stressful situations. Maeve, who is in recovery from alcohol misuse, always attends an AA meeting before going to a high-risk event and has a planned check-in call with her sponsor afterward.

BE A KID AGAIN

Lastly, a great way to reduce your overall stress load is to engage in creative outlets or activities that you enjoyed in your youth. One of my biggest joys in life is cooking. It puts me in a meditative state where I'm structured, ritualized, and focused. It also brings up fond child-hood memories of cooking with my grandmother and in kindergarten at the Montessori school. I loved to make pizza bites and sugar cookies! Perhaps you love to paint, write, play a musical instrument, sing, explore history, do photography, do improv, or travel. Maybe you want to learn a new skill, language, hobby, or take a master class to engage that childlike wonder. Your personal development domain helps you grow as an individual, reduces stress, and brings joy to your life.

9 | INTENTIONAL SLEEP

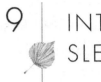

Sleep is an investment in the energy you need to be effective tomorrow.

—Robert Glazer

I'VE ALWAYS BEEN jealous of my dogs and their effortless sleep. My Bernese mountain dog, Bella, used to get up stretching, looking fully rested every morning. Whereas I often woke up at 2 a.m. and stared at the clock. Since I was a child, I have struggled with my sleep. I would wake up from a disturbing dream afraid that a monster lived in my closet. In adulthood I awaken stressing about my multiple work tasks or personal struggles that occupy my mind. It wasn't until a sleep doctor explained to me the importance of a bedtime routine that I began to appreciate how my nighttime habits were hindering my sleep.

Many busy professionals struggle with their sleep hygiene. Beth often has too much on her mind to fall asleep. Al wakes up in the middle of the night thinking about his upcoming day. Sandra admits that she burns the candle at both ends and does not make time for sleep. In fact, many professional clients routinely voice to me that they are too busy to sleep. They do not appreciate how much it impacts their careers and other life domains.

Sleep plays a vital role in optimizing overall wellness. Humans cannot function at full capacity when they are not getting enough sleep. Healthy adults need seven to nine hours of quality sleep each night.[44] When people routinely miss out on sleep, their cognition is impaired. When an individual is not as alert, it impacts safety and leads to bad personal and professional decision-making.[45] For example, Ben missed an important work deadline after a few days of unrest. Alice ran a red light on her way to the office and caused a car crash. Carter struggled with his grades in graduate school when he stayed up all night studying instead of resting before an exam.

Sleepless nights also greatly increase stress levels and may cause individuals to become moody and emotionally dysregulated. Mental health concerns like depression and anxiety also become elevated.[46] For example, Diego notices that his anxiety levels are often elevated and his mood fluctuates. Madeline craves high-calorie sugary and starchy foods. Kelsey often snaps at her husband about household responsibilities and picks trivial fights.

Moreover, disrupted sleep impacts hormone health, immunity, weight, and can put individuals at risk for developing chronic diseases.[47] Ever wonder why your internist questions you about sleep at your yearly physical exam? Bottom line, sleep is necessary to live a healthy and harmonious life.

The best way to guarantee a good night's rest is to create a bedtime routine. It all starts by choosing a consistent sleep schedule. Designate a set bedtime and rise time. This helps set your circadian rhythm, the internal process that regulates your sleep-wake cycle.[48] Try to stick with this routine even on weekends. Include an hour of bedtime wind-down. Use the following strategies to craft your own bedtime routine.

- Your bed is a sacred space. Use it for sleeping, intimacy, and your wind-down routine. Ideally, do not watch TV, talk on the phone, or do work in bed.

- Do not drink caffeine after 2 p.m. or it may result in a restless night.[49]

- Avoid large late-night meals. It's best to let the digestive system rest during the night—ideally for twelve hours—so the body can focus on repair.

- A consistent exercise routine does help you fall asleep more quickly and improves your overall sleep quality. But generally, you may want to avoid strenuous exercise later in the day.[50]

- Keep in mind that alcohol is not a sleep aid. It takes the body time to process alcohol, and although it might help an individual fall asleep, it will increase the likelihood of waking up restless during the night. Alcohol also exasperates anxiety for some individuals.[51]

- Keep the bedroom cool and dark. Cool temperatures induce sleep and result in better-quality sleep.

- Create a bedtime wind-down to relax the body and mind. Personally, I like to take a lavender detox bath, drink sleepy time tea, and then read a good book. Other wind-down ideas include:

  ★ Take a shower or bath before bedtime to cool off the body.

  ★ Complete your dental and skin-care routine.

Even when you are tired, it is important to wash your face in the evening to remove impurities (i.e., dirt, oil, bacteria, pollutants, makeup) and repair your skin.

★ Put away and turn off all electronic devices at least an hour before bedtime. While this habit may be challenging to break, electronic devices give off blue light, which disrupts sleep patterns.[52] Blue light does not allow your melatonin level to rise. (Melatonin is the hormone that regulates your sleep-wake cycle, and it naturally increases when it becomes dark outside.) You can also use the "night shift" option on your device that adjusts the color from blues to warmer colors, which can lessen the blue light emitted. Also, if this is difficult for you, start by going technology-free for ten minutes before bed and increase the time from there.

★ Read a book, journal, listen to soothing music, meditate, practice gratitude, or engage in breath work.

★ Drink herbal tea like chamomile, peppermint, ginger, or a sleepy time variety.

★ Add lavender to your nighttime routine. Lavender is a common herb used for improving sleep and reducing stress in the body. You can take a lavender detox bath for twenty minutes (2 cups Epsom salt, 1 cup baking soda, and 8–10 drops lavender essential oil), diffuse it in your room, spray it on your pillow (add a few drops of lavender essential oil to water in a spray bottle), or drink it as a tea. You can also purchase a sachet, blanket, neck pillow, or stuffed animal that contains dried lavender and heat it up in the microwave. I use a blanket that really does soothe me to sleep.

• Consult with a health-care provider about supplementation, such as melatonin, valerian, CBD oil, or other medications.

• Listen to white noise or a sound machine. White noise from a sound machine, a fan, or an app on your phone can help you fall asleep and stay asleep because it masks other noises (i.e., a door slamming, outside traffic, a spouse snoring/moving) that may stimulate the brain. Some individuals may alternatively enjoy listening to sounds of nature like the ocean, forest, or rainstorms.

- If you wake up during the night and still cannot fall back asleep after twenty minutes, get up and go to a different space to do a calming activity (read, meditate, listen to music). Remember, it's normal for some people to wake up during the night, so don't stare at the alarm clock and stress about it.

  ★ If you have too much on your mind, write a brain dump in a journal to clear your head.

- Keep track of sleep patterns by using an electronic device or keep a sleep journal. This will help determine if certain foods, activities, or occurrences assist or disrupt sleep patterns.

Additionally, when you wake up in the morning, set yourself up for success.

- Wake up to your favorite music or a pleasant alarm sound. Research has shown it is better to wake up to sounds that make you feel good rather than startled.[53]

- Stop hitting the Snooze button. When you hit the Snooze button, you drift back into sleep after waking up, which can cause you to feel groggy and exhausted for hours. It disrupts your body's internal clock. Also, the more times you press Snooze, the more likely you are to oversleep. Keep your alarm clock/phone out of reach on the other side of the room. Get up and out of bed immediately and repeat this mantra or statement three times: "feet on the floor."

- Open the curtains and take in the natural light right when you get out of bed. This will help you feel more awake and regulate your circadian rhythm. Weather permitting, step outside for a few minutes.

- Start your morning routine!

When it comes to sleep, it's all about shifting your mindset. While it might be tempting to burn the midnight oil catching up on work or zoning out on a favorite television show, you will pay the price the next day. Support your wheel of harmony by making sleep a nonnegotiable boundary you keep with yourself.

SLEEP REFLECTION

ACTION ITEM:
BEDTIME WIND-DOWN ROUTINE

What is your consistent bedtime? _____

What habits will you engage in to promote a good night's sleep?

Habit 1: _____

Habit 2: _____

Habit 3: _____

KEEP A SLEEP JOURNAL

A sleep journal may be a helpful tool for tracking sleep and any factors that might be contributing to sleep disturbances. A sleep journal identifies bedtime habits and substances that might be interfering with your sleep. Keep a sleep journal for a minimum of one week, but aim for two to three weeks. The idea is to give yourself data. Use a journal or notepad that you keep next to your bed.

In the morning, note:

- Time you went to bed

- Time you woke up

- Number of hours you slept

- Number of times you woke up

- How long it took you to fall asleep

- The quality of your sleep (i.e., excellent, good, average, bad, very poor)

- How you feel in the morning upon waking (i.e., refreshed, tired, groggy, alert)

- Anything that may have contributed to restless sleep (i.e., temperature, noise, dreams, thoughts, discomfort)

- Positive intention for the day

Before bedtime, note:

- If you took a nap during the day

- How many cups of caffeine you consumed and when

- How many minutes you exercised and when

- Any medications, drugs, or supplements you took

- Overall energy throughout the day (i.e., tired, energetic, average)

- Overall mood throughout the day (i.e., positive, negative, neutral)

- In the hour before bedtime, what activities did you engage in (i.e., reading, computer, TV, showering, eating)

- One win you had today

- Five things that you are grateful for

PART III

SET YOURSELF UP FOR SUCCESS

10 | SMART GOAL SETTING

If you fail to plan,
you are planning to fail.

—Benjamin Franklin

Winners often have a sort of secret sauce that contributes to their success. My father's is his ability to get things done; he's a master at strategic planning. For instance, when he works on a legal case, he crafts a detailed action plan, anticipating hurdles that may arise. He seeks out experts and resources and appreciates that timing matters. In a word, he's a planner.

As I've worked with clients on their wheel of harmony, I've learned it helps to create goals with this planning mindset. By planning well, we can maintain the motivation to be successful, even when hiccups arise.

When individuals fail to meet their goals, it's often because they failed to plan. For example, each year Annie sets a goal as her New Year's resolution to shift her dietary pattern. She may stay on track for a few weeks, but by Valentine's Day her motivation fades. Soon she's out of alignment with her wheel of harmony. This scenario is very common. Maybe you can relate.

Individuals benefit when they develop a strategic action plan with a clear rationale behind it. Successful corporations often follow this practice. While individuals optimize this tactic in their organization, they don't always recognize its value in their personal lives.

SMART is an acronym that helps us set and achieve goals using five anchoring words.[54] With the SMART method, you'll create attainable goals with planning that helps you achieve them. Specifically, SMART goals are *specific, measurable, achievable, relevant,* and *time bound.* SMART goals may be macro, like spending more time with family, or definitive, like completing a marathon.

SPECIFIC

SMART goals are specific and clearly defined. It's important to consider your core values and flesh out the rationale behind your goal as it relates to that value. This provides you with the intrinsic motivation vital for lasting change. For example, Ken was motivated to enhance his self-care after he experienced burnout at work and was diagnosed with depression. He knew self-care was vital to the value of enriching the relationships component of his wheel of harmony.

Reflect on the following questions:

- What do you want to accomplish?

- Why do you want to accomplish this?

- What will you gain from accomplishing it?

MEASURABLE

Lifestyle initiatives are easier to follow through on when we have a strategy to consistently monitor progress. Recording data boosts motivation and provides account-ability. Choose a measurement method like a paper tracker, spreadsheet, or smartphone app—whatever seems most doable for you. Alison keeps a habit tracker on her desk and marks off her progress each day with a star sticker.

Consider these questions:

- How will you track your progress?

- What tools will you use to measure your success (journal, phone app, spreadsheet, sales, medical test)?

- What benchmarks will help motivate you, and what will the end point be, if any?

ACHIEVABLE

Achieve your SMART goals by leaning into your daily routines and lifestyle habits. Designate three lifestyle habits and map out three strategies to help you successfully achieve them. You have a whole tool kit of strategies from the self-care chapters. These initiatives should be built into morning, evening, workday, and exercise routines. For instance, Rob created the habit of sleeping seven to nine hours per night as part of his overarching SMART goal of improving his self-care. He planned to achieve this by using the following strategies: setting a consistent sleep schedule, forgoing electronic devices an hour before bedtime, and reading a book.

Achievable goals require planning. Consider hurdles that may prevent you from following through. We are creatures of habit. Unwanted behaviors will try to creep back in. Therefore, set yourself up to succeed by planning in advance what you'll do when hurdles arise. For instance, Rob misses out on sleep when he binges on streaming services. He guards against this by setting an evening notification on his smartphone at his designated wind-down time. Also, identify the people in your life who can support you and communicate your goals to them.[55]

Ask yourself these questions:

- How will you accomplish this goal?

- What three habits will you build into your routine to accomplish this goal?

- What three strategies will you use to build out each habit, specifically in the morning, evening, and during workdays versus the weekend?

- What hurdles do you anticipate?

- Who will support you?

RELEVANT

A SMART goal can realistically be achieved given your current life circumstances. So focus on something that is attainable at this moment in time. For example, Maggie is about to start a three-month trial away from home, so joining her neighborhood gym won't help her achieve fitness goals as she will not be around to make use of it. She will need to strategize another avenue to jump-start her fitness plan.

Ask yourself these questions:

- Does this goal align with your values?

- Does this goal align with your availability, finances, and resources?

- Does this goal enhance the quality of your wheel of harmony?

TIME BOUND

Finally, SMART goals are time bound. When you assign a specific ending date, you'll be motivated and able to easily evaluate progress. Some goals build on each other over time, while others may be broken down into smaller time increments. For example, Adam wanted to lose thirty pounds, but he broke it into smaller increments, starting with a ten-pound weight loss goal over three months. He found this achievable and believed meeting it would spur his motivation.

Smaller, achievable wins build momentum. Celebrate successes big and small. Reward yourself with a massage, new workout shoes, concert tickets, or even a family vacation. When a goal is time bound, you can celebrate as soon as that goal is reached.

Ask yourself these questions:

- What is the time frame for accomplishing your goal? One month? Two? Six?

- Is this time frame realistic for you?

- What will you do to celebrate your win?

NECESSARY BOUNDARIES

Having set your SMART goals, revisit your list of boundaries from chapter 3 to determine if any boundaries need to be in place to guarantee success in achieving your SMART goals. For example, Randy, who wants to exercise three times a week, plans to log his sessions as a recurrence in his calendar and schedule work meetings around them. That way he will guard against scheduling on top of his priority.

EVALUATING PROGRESS
OVER TIME

It's important to evaluate your progress after your time allotment ends for your SMART goal. If you feel confident in your SMART goal accomplishment, consider how you want to proceed. You may want to set a new SMART goal highlighting additional avenues for self-care or choose another life domain to enhance your wheel of harmony.

"Failure is just data." I like this quote because it reminds me that if something does not work, it's just an opportunity. Think of it as knowledge gained. Use it to either tweak your SMART goal or reset your focus. For example, Laura set a SMART goal that included the habit of meditating thirty minutes per day. When she evaluated her progress, she saw that after the first month she started missing days of meditation. Why? Thirty minutes felt too overwhelming. She reset her SMART goal to five to ten minutes of meditation per day and was successful.

Build on small, doable changes over time. As you accomplish SMART goals, maintain the lifestyle initiatives that are working for you. Over time, this will create long-term fulfillment in your wheel of harmony.

SMART GOAL CASE STUDY

Let's revisit Jenny from chapter 2. Here's how she used the SMART acronym to flesh out her plan.

Specific: I will improve my health by making my self-care a top priority. I am committed to creating more harmony in my life so I can enjoy precious time with my family and be at my best to achieve my career goals.

Measurable: I am going to get my blood work retested in six months and track my daily habits in a journal.

Achievable: I will improve my health and self-care by engaging in the following consistent habits:

HABIT 1: Exercise three times a week.

- Schedule it in my calendar.

- Pack my gym and work clothes the night before.

- Work out with my friend as an accountability partner.

HABIT 2: Practice mindfulness for stress management.

- Download a meditation app on my smartphone.

- Dedicate a place in my home for meditation.

- Practice as part of my bedtime wind-down routine.

HABIT 3: Eat five homemade meals a week with my family.

- Grocery shop and meal prep on Sundays.

- Each week let one family member pick a theme night and build a healthy meal around it—Italian, Greek, Taco Tuesday, Meatless Monday.

- Create a family rule to have no smartphones at the dinner table.

I anticipate the following hurdles:

- Failing to grocery shop and meal prep and then ordering carryout on the way home from work for dinner.

- Making excuses to skip scheduled exercise—"I'm too tired" or "I don't have enough time."

- Staying up late to binge a television show instead of engaging in my bedtime routine.

Relevant: I value my family and health, but I have gotten out of alignment with my self-care and values. These new habits are doable for me with my lifestyle, and my family is supportive.

Time Bound: I will revisit my goal at my doctor's appointment in six months. My family is also planning a tropical vacation to celebrate progress together.

I will enforce the following necessary boundaries.

- I will not schedule work meetings during my allotted exercise time.

- My family will place phones in a basket before dinner.

- I will remove the television from the bedroom.

ACTION ITEM: SMART GOAL

Now that you have built a solid foundation and have a clear direction for your wheel of harmony, it's time to create an action plan. Start by setting one SMART goal to focus on. Your SMART goal should be guided by your values and reflect your life domains of focus. Weave your self-care routines into your action plan and set necessary boundaries to ensure success.

Specific: _____

_____

_____

Measurable: _____

_____

_____

_____

Achievable: _____

_____

_____

_____

Habit: _____

Strategy 1: _____

Strategy 2: _____

Strategy 3: _____

Habit: _____

Strategy 1: _____

Strategy 2: _____

Strategy 3: _____

Habit: _____

Strategy 1: _____

Strategy 2: _____

Strategy 3: _____

Anticipated Hurdles: _____

_____

Relevant: _____

_____

_____

Time Bound: _____

_____

_____

11 | TROUBLE-SHOOTING DURING BUSY SEASONS

Self-care is not a waste of time.
Self-care makes your use of time
more sustainable.

—JACKIE VIRAMONTEZ

A CORE PRINCIPLE of this book is *harmony*. I use that word rather than *balance* because there is really no such thing as balance. We all experience busy seasons where maintaining routine is just unrealistic. Like the weeks when I'm traveling to conferences, or when life seems so hectic that working out and cooking homemade meals is completely unfeasible. This is when I give myself grace and adjust to accommodate my current life circumstances.

There are many ways to pivot during stressful

periods. For example, when Maggie is on trial, she has healthy meals and snacks delivered to her office. After Henry's wife had surgery, he adjusted his work schedule to care for her and the family. When Gina travels, she tracks her steps instead of completing her planned workouts. Even in periods of stress, the stress is manageable when we intentionally modify regular routines to accommodate our values and priorities. Use the following strategies to troubleshoot.

WORK TRAVEL

Work travel can take a mental and physical toll. Individuals may face sleep disruptions and limited access to healthy meals and exercise facilities. There may also be inadequate time for self-care and a lack of boundaries. Not to mention all the stress associated with travel—airports, delays, sitting for long periods, tension with colleagues, problems at home. While mindful planning won't eliminate all stressors, planning will allow you to feel deliberate alignment in your wheel of harmony.

BOOK YOUR HOTEL WITH A SPECIAL REQUEST AND IDENTIFY HEALTHY FOOD OPTIONS

People now have access at their fingertips to researching healthy options when they are away from home. For instance, when Lupe travels, she requests a microwave and refrigerator for her hotel room. She finds grocery stores close to the hotel and orders healthy food to be delivered.

Individuals can use the fridge to store fresh produce and ingredients for easy meal prep. Fast and healthy microwavable meals include oatmeal, an egg scramble (use a coffee mug, throw in some veggies), and frozen meals that include lean protein, veggies, and a carb. Stock up on nutritious and balanced snacks—hummus and carrots, yogurt and berries, nut butter and whole-grain crackers, string cheese and apple. This will keep you energized throughout the day and less tempted to order late-night room service.

RESEARCH EXERCISE OPTIONS

Many hotels have twenty-four-hour gyms or offer special day rates at nearby fitness centers. When Sam travels, he is often able to find his franchised studio and use his membership to take a class. Lucy loves to map out running trails before she goes on a business trip, and Kenneth always books hotels with a lap pool. I bring my exercise bands with me and work out in my hotel room with one of my favorite apps. When all else fails, walk to a meeting or restaurant instead of taking the rideshare.

BE PREPARED FOR TRAVEL DAYS

Travel with healthy snacks or buy some from convenience stores—nuts or trail mix, protein bars, beef jerky, string cheese, Greek yogurt, hard-boiled eggs. You can even request meals on many flights. Be prepared to keep your mind occupied. You'll reduce travel anxiety and make good use of delays by catching up on work, reading, or enjoying podcasts, shows, or movies.

DINING OUT

Check restaurant menus online before going out and commit to a healthy meal choice. Jane, who regularly tracks her meals, preplans her dining out meals in the app and then bases the rest of her day's nutrition around them. Always lead with the protein option, and don't be afraid to ask the server for a different meal preparation. Consider ordering an appetizer as a main course or eat half your main dish and save the remainder for the following day. Further, watch alcohol intake. Overconsumption can lead to unhealthy food choices, loss of sleep, and increased anxiety.

STRESS MANAGEMENT FOR BUSY SEASONS

During busy periods, it may be tempting to abandon wellness routines and SMART goal action plans until things slow down. This will only create a vicious cycle. Life keeps moving and there will always be something. It's precisely during these stressful periods that you need self-care practices to thrive.

GOLDEN RULE: SOMETHING IS ALWAYS BETTER THAN NOTHING

Instead of abandoning routines during busy seasons, remember that something is always better than nothing. If you can't fit it all in, find ways to modify your routines and incorporate self-care pockets. Little wins here and there add up.

- Pause in your day to do breath work or a meditation exercise.

- Take the stairs instead of the elevator.

- Walk to an appointment.

- Do a ten-minute workout on an app.

- Do a set of planks, push-ups, sit-ups,
  or jumping jacks.

- After a long day, enjoy a cup of chamomile tea
  instead of a cocktail.

- Read a book at night as opposed to getting
  on your laptop.

- Order a side salad instead of the fries.

- Be mindful about staying hydrated throughout
  the day.

- Stretch before bed.

MAKE SLEEP A MUST

Do not underestimate the value of sleep. Even if you cannot get your desired seven to nine hours of quality sleep, still strive to get at least six hours. Human beings need time to recharge. You need the energy and mental clarity sleep provides for the next day's grind.

EAT TO BOOST MOOD AND MANAGE ANXIETY

When I was in graduate school, I did my capstone research project on how to use nutrition as a tool to reduce and manage depression and anxiety disorders. The research supports following a Mediterranean-focused diet of nutrient-dense foods.[56] Further studies indicate that individuals benefit from reducing their consumption of Omega-6 vegetable oils, sweeteners, and caffeine.[57] Therefore, individuals prone to anxiety and depression benefit greatly from increasing their consumption of the following nutritional gems:

MOOD BOOSTERS[58]

- Omega-3 polyunsaturated fatty acids (PUFAs)—salmon, tuna, flaxseeds, walnuts, chia seeds

- Kale and other leafy greens and lettuces

- Cruciferous vegetables—broccoli, cauliflower, cabbage, brussels sprouts

- Seafood and organ meats

ANXIETY REDUCERS

- Omega-3 polyunsaturated fatty acids (PUFAs)—salmon, tuna, flaxseeds, walnuts, chia seeds[59]

- Probiotics—yogurt, kefir, sauerkraut, pickles, miso, and kimchi[60]

- Choline—eggs, meat, liver, soybeans[61]

- Gluten-free whole grains—quinoa, wild rice, oats[62]

- Reduce caffeine[63]

See appendix B for a mood-boosting meal plan and recipe guide. This meal plan is meant as a reference guide to assist you in bringing some new foods and flavors into your home. The snack suggestions are also a great way for you to boost your mood and energy during the busy workday.

TAKE A REAL VACATION

Many professionals admit reluctance to use their vacation time or have difficulty leaving work behind. These are legitimate fears that stem from being a part of a work culture that has high expectations and values performance. For instance, when Frank vacations with his family, he routinely feels the urge to check his work email. To live in harmony across your life areas, it's important to recharge your body, mind, and spirit. Reboot in those areas and you'll be more productive in your life domains *and* foster fulfillment. After all, making memories by visiting new places is one of the most joyful experiences in life. I will never forget the magical experience I had exploring Viennese Christmas markets with my husband and parents on a recent vacation.

Use the following strategies to unplug and lessen any anxieties that may arise around using your vacation time:

- Communicate with your colleagues and clients in advance about your absence. Supply plans and instructions to anyone covering your work.

- Establish clear boundaries with clients and coworkers about your availability and what type of urgency will constitute an "emergency" call or email.

- Commit to unplugging by turning off work email notifications and texts. If you feel it is necessary to regularly check your work communications, designate a window of time each day and maintain this boundary with yourself.

- Give yourself permission to relax. Use time away to enjoy the location, moment, and the company you are with. Life is short and you cannot get these experiences back.

- If your schedule or circumstances do not allow for a formal vacation, take a staycation—and enjoy it as if you were away.

PLAN RESET WEEKS

Don't beat yourself up if you get off track. It happens. The whole purpose of creating routines is so you have a solid base to return to when life gets in the way of self-care. Designate a week to make wellness a top priority. Reengage with your daily routines and clear the calendar of any unnecessary events. For example, when Suzanne returns home from a conference, she uses the following week to catch up on work and prioritizes self-care. She also maintains her boundaries by declining social obligations.

Schedule reset weeks to intentionally give yourself grace and create your plan to get back on track and realign with your wheel of harmony.

CONCLUSION:
SLOW AND STEADY WINS THE WELLNESS RACE

Slow and steady wins the race.

—A PROVERB

I HAVE ALWAYS loved the famous Aesop fable "The Tortoise and the Hare." The Hare thought he would easily win the competition because he moved more swiftly. So much so that during the race, he lay down on the side of the course to take a nap. Meanwhile, the Tortoise kept moving along slowly and steadily, passing the sleeping Hare and winning the race.

While it may be tempting to speed ahead like the Hare, slow and steady does win the wellness race. Life is a marathon, not a sprint. When people make changes or decisions too quickly, they often burn out. Fully consider big life changes before leaning into new life-style initiatives.

A fun way to stay motivated in your wheel of harmony is by creating a personal mantra that aligns with your SMART goals. A mantra is a phrase or statement that encourages positive self-talk.[64] Your interpretation of yourself and the situation is what gives it meaning. Become empowered by living your personal mantra and practicing it every day.

For example, every morning Gretchen says, "I am a beautiful, confident, and perfectly imperfect woman."

Patrick notes, "I am an active man, and my health is a top priority."

Kellyanne states, "I live according to my wheel of harmony and prioritize self-care."

Al voices, "I am committing to boundaries because I want to protect the things that are important to me."

Write a personal mantra here._____

_____

_____

_____

Practice your mantra by saying it aloud. Every day look in the bathroom mirror and say your mantra aloud (or in your head) as part of your routine. Keep it posted somewhere you'll see it often, like your bathroom mirror, vehicle visor, workstation, wallet, or refrigerator. Revisit your mantra as inspiration anytime you need a mental boost.

Another way to stay engaged with your mantra is to choose a totem. It can be an animal, object, emblem, piece of clothing, jewelry, picture, or screen saver that has significant meaning to you. Currently, my mantra is a butterfly because I've done a lot of transforming in committing to live my wheel of harmony. For me, the butterfly represents that intention.

Layne, who feels like he planted roots in his new role as a father, connects with the totem of an oak tree. Jenny's totem is a photo of her family representing her whys. Change up your mantras and totems as you craft new SMART goals and begin new chapters in your life.

What is your totem? _____

_____

_____

Congratulations on completing your wellness adventure! I hope this book inspired you to design a wheel of harmony uniquely authentic to you, guided by your values and supportive of self-care. It has been my honor to be your guide on this exploration. You have all the tools you need to live a harmonious, fulfilling life. Please revisit this book when you need a refresher or a reset.

BE WELL.

APPENDIX A
MEAL PLANNING GUIDE

KEEPING YOUR KITCHEN stocked with staples will make your meal planning much easier and give you lots of ways to create flavorful meals in a pinch. Experiment and add staples to your tool kit that you and your family enjoy.

FATS AND OILS:

Grass-fed butter, extra-virgin olive oil, avocado oil, coconut oil, ghee, grapeseed oil (flavorless), sesame oil, walnut oil, MCT oil

VINEGARS:

Apple cider vinegar, balsamic vinegar, rice vinegar, red wine vinegar, white wine vinegar

ADD-INS AND CONDIMENTS:

Dijon mustard, gluten-free soy sauce or coconut aminos, Worcestershire sauce, mayonnaise, tomato paste, pesto, siracha or hot sauce

SWEETENERS:

Honey, maple syrup, monk fruit sweetener, sugar, raw stevia, or coconut sugar

SEASONINGS:

Kosher salt, sea salt, black pepper, oregano, thyme, turmeric, chili powder, cayenne, Ceylon cinnamon, cumin, fresh parsley, fresh basil, fresh cilantro, red pepper flakes, rosemary, sage, paprika, dill. Spice stores often have essential spice collections.

PROTEINS:

Eggs, grass-fed beef, tempeh or extra-firm tofu, chicken, ground turkey breast, nitrate-free bacon or turkey bacon, shrimp, canned tuna or wild salmon, dried or canned beans, lentils, hummus

GRAINS:

Brown rice, wild rice, basmati rice, rolled oats, quinoa, barley, cornmeal, whole grain pastas, gluten-free pastas (brown rice, lentil, quinoa, chickpea, cassava)

NUTS AND SEEDS:

Nut butters, tahini, almonds, walnuts, Brazil nuts,

cashews, macadamia nuts, pistachios, pumpkin seeds, sesame seeds, flaxseeds, chia seeds

DAIRY AND DAIRY ALTERNATIVES:

Unsweetened Greek yogurt, coconut, almond or cashew milks and yogurts, feta cheese, Parmesan cheese, cheddar cheese, string cheese, cream cheese

AROMATICS:

Scallions, fresh ginger, garlic, onions (red, white, or yellow), carrots, celery, leeks

NON-STARCHY VEGETABLES:

Artichokes, artichoke hearts, asparagus, bamboo shoots, bean sprouts, beets, broccoli, brussels sprouts, cabbage (green, bok choy, Chinese), cauliflower, celery, cucumber, daikon, eggplant, fennel, leeks, lentils, leafy greens (arugula, butter lettuce, chicory, collard, endive, escarole, iceberg lettuce, kale, mustard, radicchio, romaine, spinach, turnip, watercress), mushrooms, okra, onions, pea pods, peppers, radishes, rutabaga, squash, sugar snap peas, Swiss chard, tomato, water chestnuts, watercress, zucchini (zoodles)

FRUITS:

Lemons, limes, avocados, fresh or frozen berries, apples, oranges, grapefruit, bananas

OTHERS:

Chicken broth, beef broth, vegetable broth, cooking wine

WEEKLY MEAL PREPPING

Your brain loves a plan. Choose a day of the week and make that your designated meal-prepping day. Some individuals like to divide the prepping into two days each week.

Supplies

• Wooden cutting board or Epicurean cutting board

• Sharpened chef knife

• Mason jars

• Glass storage containers or BPA-free plastic storage containers

• Tinfoil

• Plastic wrap

- Ziplock bags

- Pots and pans, baking sheets, bench scraper, cooking utensils (i.e., wooden spoons, spatulas, graters, peelers, meat thermometers) and baking utensils (i.e., measuring cups, mixing bowls, muffin tins, rolling pin)

- Optional appliances: high-quality blender, immersion blender, food processor, hand mixer, stand mixer, slow cooker, Instant Pot, air fryer, grill

Planning

- Plan out your meals for the week. Remember, leftovers work great for lunch or another meal.

- Consider if you will be dining out and factor this into your schedule.

- Write everything down on a calendar or whiteboard in your kitchen.

- Create a grocery list of ingredients that you need. Note that you should shop in your pantry, refrigerator, and freezer first. For instance, you may already have frozen chicken breasts, canned tuna, or wild rice.

- Go to the grocery store or call a delivery service (i.e., Instacart, Amazon Prime, Pea Pod, Thrive Market).

- You can also use a meal kit or prepared meals delivery service (i.e., Sun Basket, Blue Apron, Home Chef, Marley Spoon, Factor).

Prepping

- Designate one day a week as your meal-prepping day.

- Wash, cut, and store your vegetables and fruits in food storage containers. Properly stored produce will last all week and make your life much easier. You can then use these vegetables and fruits in salads, as snack options, or as a side dish roasted, steamed, or sautéed.

- Prep protein options, such as grilled chicken breasts, quinoa, tuna salad, hard-boiled eggs, and beans.

- Prep full meals two to three days ahead of cooking, such as a meat loaf, casserole, or stuffed peppers.

Helpful Hints

- While you are preparing dinner, pack your lunch and snacks and prep your breakfast for the following morning.

- Always have a go-to meal readily available for breakfast, lunch, and dinner, such as frozen crustless quiches, chili, casseroles, frozen healthy dinners, and soups.

- Buy extra meat or fish when it's on sale and store it in plastic baggies in individual or family-sized portions in your freezer.

- Have cookbooks, websites, and recipe apps book-marked for quick reference.

- Create a master list of all the meals in your repertoire that you enjoy.

YOUR FREEZER IS YOUR FRIEND

A great way to have healthy meals on hand is to double a recipe and freeze the second batch. You can also make freezer-friendly meals.

Supplies

- Ziplock freezer bags

- Tinfoil

- Plastic wrap

- Disposable foil pans

Freezer Tips

- Let foods cool completely before freezing them to avoid freezer burn. Ideally, completely refrigerate foods before freezing to prevent ice crystals from forming on top.

- Freeze foods flat in ziplock freezer bags to avoid clumping. This will also allow you to stack them easily.

- Chop fruits and vegetables before freezing and lay flat in a ziplock freezer bag.

- Remove as much air as possible from freezer bags before freezing.

- Label bags/packaging with the date frozen, enjoy-by date, contents, and reheating instructions.

- Wrap foods that don't fit in freezer bags, like breads, first in plastic wrap and then foil.

- If using plastic or glass containers to freeze liquids like broth or soup, leave room at the top for liquid to expand once frozen.

According to the National Center for Home Food Preservation, the following are monthly storage estimates for foods. Note that the sooner you eat the food or meal, the fresher it will be.

- **Fruits and Vegetables:** 8–12 months

- **Poultry:** 6–9 months

- **Fish:** 3–6 months

- **Ground Meat:** 3–4 months

- **Cured or Processed Meat:** 1–2 months

HOW TO BEST FREEZE AND REHEAT BASIC MEALS

- **Soups, Stews, and Chili:** Chill completely, scoop into gallon ziplock bags, and freeze flat. Thaw overnight in the refrigerator, then reheat in a pot on the stove.

- **Sauces:** Chill completely, scoop into gallon ziplock bags, and freeze flat. Thaw overnight in the refrigerator, then reheat in a saucepan.

- **Meats:** You can freeze burgers, steaks, chicken, meat loaf, and meatballs cooked or uncooked in freezer bags. Thaw meat in the refrigerator, then bake/

prepare according to recipe instructions. When freezing cooked ground meat, cool cooked meat completely and then transfer to a freezer bag and freeze flat.

- **Casseroles:** Assemble casseroles up to the baking step in a foil pan, cover tightly with plastic wrap and then foil, and freeze. Thaw in the refrigerator overnight, then bake according to recipe instructions.

- **Breads, Muffins, and Crustless Quiche:** For breads, cool completely and then wrap in plastic wrap and freeze in a ziplock freezer bag (or wrap in foil if they won't fit in a bag). For muffins and crustless quiche, first freeze on a sheet pan, then transfer to a freezer bag. Thaw in the refrigerator or on the counter, or wrap in paper towels while frozen and microwave at 50 percent power until warm.

- **Herbs and Pesto:** Ice cube containers are a great way to preserve herbs (freeze in water) or pesto sauces.

HEALTHY RECIPE HACKS

Being healthy should not mean sacrificing fun and flavor. Here are simple hacks to *healthify* your meals:

- **Sneak** in vegetables for breakfast—smoothies and egg dishes are simple meals that allow you to add in a variety of vegetables

- **Swap** pasta for spaghetti squash and zoodles or substitute for half

- **Replace** heavy cream with unsweetened coconut cream or unsweetened nut milk (i.e., almond, cashew), oat milk, or use 1/2 cream and 1/2 broth

- **Use** alternative flours for dredging, breadcrumbs, and baking—almond flour, cassava flour, white rice flour, tapioca flour, and coconut flour

- **Replace** bread with vegetables—use portobello mushrooms, sweet potato medallions, and Boston lettuce leaves

- **Use** mason jars for meals-on-the-go and storage

- **Make** homemade desserts with fruits and vegetables

- **Cook** healthy sheet tray meals in a jiff

10 VEGETABLE PREPARATION IDEAS

- **Blend** into smoothies

- **Steam** and serve with dressing or drizzle with tamari and sesame oil or with olive oil and lemon

- **Roast** with olive oil, grapeseed oil, garlic, and herbs (400 degrees) and top with roasted nuts (pine nuts, almonds, walnuts)

- **Sauté** with olive oil and garlic/onions, coconut oil

- **Stir-fry** with ginger, scallions, or garlic

- **Grill** with grapeseed oil, salt, and pepper. Drizzle balsamic vinegar on top

- **Mash** cauliflower or carrots

- **Blanch** kale, dark leafy greens, or collard greens in boiling salted water (2–3 minutes) and then **sauté** with olive oil and seasoning

- **Sneak** vegetables into your meals by chopping finely and adding to tomato sauces and soups

- **Use a micro plane** for grating on extra flavor (lemon zest, orange zest, lime zest, garlic, ginger)

CONSOLIDATE COOKING

Make the most of your time in the kitchen by making double the amount of basic foods. Serve one way the first night and then use the rest for another meal.

Beans and Soy

- Serve as a side dish

- Use as a base for stir-fry

- Add to soup

- Add to salad

- Add to a whole grain or pasta dish

- Puree into a spread

- Taco filling

- Tostada topping

- Add to taco salad

- Burrito filling

Eggs

- Frittata

- Scramble

- Egg salad

- Omelet with your favorite veggies

- Hard-boil extra and add to green salads
  or make egg salad

Fish and Poultry (Baked, Roasted, or Grilled)

- Shred and add to BBQ sauce for burger
  or wrap filling

- Serve as an entrée

- Add to salad

- Add to veggies for fajita filling

- Add to stir-fry veggies

- Shred for burrito filling

- Add to whole grains or pasta

- Slice for sandwiches

- Add to soup

- Cook a double batch and freeze half

Rice or Whole Grains

- Serve as an entrée with sauce

- Use as a base for stir-fry

- Mix with beans for a burrito

- Add to soup

- Make rice pudding

- Serve as a side dish

- Toss with olive oil and garlic for a side dish

- Make a whole grain or pasta salad toss. Toss with sun-dried tomatoes, artichokes, olives, mozzarella, and basil.

HOUSEHOLD MEAL-PREPPING IDEAS:

The Individual

- Invest in a mini slow cooker or small Instant Pot

- Eat leftovers for lunch

- Repurpose your leftovers into entirely different meals

- If leftover food is not your jam, store all your prepped foods individually so you can mix them in different meal combinations

- Create a stockpile of frozen meals so you can have a different dinner every night

- Avoid buying prepackaged meats and produce and buy amounts you will use (or freeze excess)

- Shop with a friend and share

The Couple

- See individual meal-prep ideas above

- Most recipes serve 4–6 people.
  Cut the ingredients in half or plan on
  freezing half for an easy weeknight meal.

- Take turns cooking dinner

- Take a cooking class together

- Have a date night

Family

- Use resources like Pinterest and Instagram for ideas

- Buy pre-prepped proteins and bags of pre-cut vegetables at the grocery store

- Cook one-pot meals, soups, and sheet tray dinners for busy weeknights

- Invest in a large Instant Pot or slow cooker

- Know your family's go-to meals and have ingredients on hand

- Make double the recipe and freeze the second recipe

- Let your family build their own dishes to accommodate everyone's needs (chili, baked potato, burger, taco bar, stir-fry, homemade pizza, salads)

- Let your children help you in the kitchen—they'll be more likely to try new things

- Use extra dinner ingredients to create flexible lunches (i.e., roast chicken dinner to a chicken wrap, bento boxes)

- Buy extra meat, fish, and produce when it is on sale

- Bulk shop (i.e., Costco, Butcher Box)

- Have each family member come up with a theme night dinner and menu

- Post the weekly menu planner on your refrigerator with instructions so anyone can start dinner

SAMPLE MEAL IDEAS

Breakfast

- Smoothie

- Yogurt and fruit

- Berry parfait with granola

- Cottage cheese and fruit

- 1 slice whole grain toast or English muffin with almond butter, cinnamon, and a sprinkle of raw walnuts (optional)

- Vegetable omelet, side of fruit

- Eggs any style on 1 slice whole grain toast and 1/2 grapefruit

- Egg and vegetable muffins (make in muffin tins with favorite combinations)

- Oatmeal with minced apples, slivered almonds, and cinnamon

- Chocolate oatmeal (add in chocolate protein powder and dairy-free milk to consistency)

- Overnight oats

- High-fiber, low-sugar cereal with milk or dairy-free

milk with fruit and ground flaxseed

- Chia seed pudding

- Protein pancakes

- Smoked salmon or turkey with tomato and onion on 1/2 whole grain bagel

- Avocado toast

Lunch or Dinner

- 4–6 oz. grilled chicken, fish, lean beef, or bison with steamed vegetables (drizzle a touch of olive oil and lemon on top); if you are having a starch at this meal: 1/2 to 1 cup whole grain (i.e., brown rice, wild rice, quinoa) or sweet potato

- Create a custom go-to salad or sandwich

- Turkey sandwich on whole grain bread, wrap, or rice cake with vegetable trimmings, condiments, side of fruit

- Turkey or veggie burger wrapped in Boston lettuce or atop 1/2 whole grain English muffin or 1/2 whole grain bun with toppings (tomato, onion, sautéed mushrooms and spinach, organic cheese, etc.) and side salad

- Vegetable frittata, side of fruit

- Soup (non-cream base) and a mixed greens salad

- Soup (non-cream base) and 1/2 sandwich or melt

- Chicken and veggie stir-fry with brown rice, cauli-flower rice, or soba noodles

- Chicken salad or tuna salad platter with a mixed greens side salad and fruit

- Chicken salad or tuna salad pita

- Chicken lettuce wraps

- Turkey or beef meat loaf with roasted vegetables

- Pesto and vegetable quesadillas

- Green salad with leftover meat or beans, fruit, nuts/ seeds, dressing (i.e., chicken atop arugula with straw-berries, walnuts, and vinaigrette)

- Quinoa bowl with vegetables

- Turkey, beef, or lentil meatballs over spaghetti (whole grain noodles, bean/lentil pasta, or zoodles)

- Lasagna

- Stuffed peppers

- Taco night

- Chili and/or baked potato bar

- Sloppy Joes

- Sheet tray chicken, salmon, or shrimp dinners

- Favorite slow cooker and Instant Pot meals

Snacks

- Chocolate banana smoothie

- Apple with 1–2 tablespoons unsweetened almond butter, cashew butter, peanut butter, or Justine's individual nut butter packs

- Fruit and piece of string cheese

- Celery sticks with 1–2 tablespoons unsweetened nut butter, unsweetened raisins, and cinnamon

- Apple, orange, or 1/2 grapefruit with 10 almonds, walnuts halves, macadamia nuts, or cashews

- 1/4 cup nuts

- Vegetable sticks with 1/3 cup hummus

- 1/2 cup tuna salad with whole grain crackers or almond flour crackers

- 1 oz. dark chocolate with 1–2 tablespoons almond butter

- 1 hard-boiled egg

- Turkey roll-ups (turkey slices, vegetables, and condiment)

- 1/4 cup guacamole or black bean dip, salsa, and serving of blue tortilla chips or grain-free tortilla chips

- 1/2 cup cottage cheese, 2/3 cup unsweetened Greek yogurt, coconut yogurt, almond yogurt, or cashew yogurt and 1 cup berries

- Chia seed pudding

- Meal replacement bar (read labels)

- Trail mix (1/4 cup serving)—make your own by mixing a combination of your favorite nuts, seeds, unsweetened dried fruit, and cacao nibs

- Kale chips

- Homemade protein balls or energy bites

- Rice cake with unsweetened nut butter

APPENDIX B
MOOD-BOOSTING MEAL PLAN AND RECIPE GUIDE

	BREAKFAST	LUNCH	SNACK	DINNER
DAY 1	Egg Muffins and Fruit	Strawberry Chicken and Arugula Salad	Beauty Protein Bites	One Pot Shrimp Scampi and Broccoli
DAY 2	Rasperry Yogurt Smoothie	Tuna Salad Platter	Roasted Kale and Pumpkin Seed Chips	Buffalo Turkey Chili and Almond Coconut Drop Biscuits
DAY 3	Pumpkin Spice Overnight Oats	Turkey Apple Wrap	Whole Grain Crackers and 1 String Cheese	Salmon with Soy Glaze, Roasted Asparagus and 1/2 Cup Wild Rice
DAY 4	Avocado Toast and Scrambled Egg with Mixed Berries	Miso Soup and Mixed Greens Side Salad	Turkey Roll-Ups	Black Bean and Quinoa Burger with Carrot and Green Bean Fries
DAY 5	Vegetable Omelet	Kale Walnut Pesto Pasta Salad	1/4 Cup Nuts and Orange	Baked Fish in Parchment Paper and Greek Lemon Potatoes
DAY 6	Blueberry Overnight Oats	Portobello Turkey Burger and Mixed Greens Side Salad	1/4 Cup Hummus and Vegetable Sticks	Free Meal
DAY 7	Berry Parfait	Simple Lentil Soup and Slice Sourdough Bread	Celery Sticks with 1 Tablespoon Unsweetened Almond Butter, Unsweetened Raisins, and Cinnamon	BBQ Sheet Tray Chicken Dinner

GROCERY LIST

Select which recipes you will be cooking this week and check off the ingredients that you need to purchase. Note that some of these foods may already be staples in your kitchen and freezer or will make great additions to your healthy pantry.

Vegetables and Leafy Greens

☐ 2 bunches kale

☐ 2 bunches or containers spinach

☐ 2 bunches or containers arugula

☐ 1 Boston lettuce head

☐ 2 red peppers

☐ 1 yellow pepper

☐ 1 cucumber

☐ 1 pound cremini or button mushrooms

☐ 8 portobello mushrooms

☐ 2 broccoli crowns

☐ 1 pound asparagus

☐ 4 yellow onions

☐ 1 red onion

☐ 1 shallot

☐ 1 bunch scallions

☐ 3 medium tomatoes

- [ ] 2 pints cherry tomatoes
- [ ] 1 large zucchini
- [ ] 1 large celery bunch
- [ ] 8 large carrots
- [ ] 3 medium russet potatoes
- [ ] 3 medium sweet potatoes
- [ ] 1 bunch green beans
- [ ] 1 bunch brussels sprouts
- [ ] 2 garlic bulbs
- [ ] 1 bunch fresh chives
- [ ] 1 bunch fresh basil
- [ ] 1 bunch fresh parsley
- [ ] 1 bunch fresh cilantro
- [ ] 1 bunch fresh rosemary
- [ ] 1 can pumpkin puree
- [ ] 1 (15 oz.) can tomato sauce
- [ ] 2 (15 oz.) can diced tomatoes
- [ ] 1 small can artichoke hearts

Fruits

- [ ] 1 bag frozen raspberries
- [ ] 1 bag frozen wild blueberries
- [ ] 1 pint fresh strawberries
- [ ] 2 cups berries or melons

☐ 3 lemons

☐ 1 avocado

☐ 1 green apple

☐ 1 orange

☐ 1 package dried cranberries

☐ 1 package dried raisins

Protein

*Note that it's always a great idea to buy meat and fish when it's on sale and freeze it for future use. You can also buy sources in bulk online on discount websites, such as the **Butcher Box**.*

☐ 1/2 pound nitrate-free deli turkey breast

☐ 8 boneless, skinless chicken breasts, divided

☐ 3 pounds ground turkey breast, divided

☐ 6 oz. water-packed tuna

☐ 2 6-oz. portions of wild salmon

☐ 4 white fish filets

☐ 1 pound shrimp, peeled and deveined

☐ 2 cartons eggs

☐ 16 oz. container Greek yogurt or unsweetened non-dairy yogurt (i.e., Kite Hill)

☐ 1 carton unsweetened almond milk or non-dairy milk

☐ Cheddar cheese or vegan cheese

- [ ] 1 small container low-fat cottage cheese
- [ ] 1 block or container Parmesan cheese
- [ ] 1 string cheese
- [ ] 1 block or container feta cheese (optional)
- [ ] 1 package firm tofu
- [ ] 1 package red lentils
- [ ] 1 (15 oz.) can chili beans in sauce
- [ ] 1 (15 oz.) can black beans

Note that the first time you go to the grocery store, you will be investing in you. These staples will last you for months. You can save money by buying online on discount websites, such as Thrive Market.

Healthy Fats
- [ ] Olive oil or avocado cooking spray
- [ ] Olive oil
- [ ] Avocado oil
- [ ] Ghee or grass-fed butter
- [ ] Coconut butter
- [ ] Coconut oil
- [ ] Sesame oil
- [ ] Chia seeds
- [ ] Ground flaxseeds

- [ ] Pumpkin seeds
- [ ] Walnuts
- [ ] Cashew butter
- [ ] Almond butter
- [ ] Nuts (i.e., almonds, cashew)

Whole Grains and Starches

- [ ] Whole wheat or spelt orzo pasta
- [ ] 1 loaf sprouted grain bread like Ezekiel or sourdough bread (store in freezer for several months)
- [ ] 1 package granola (i.e., Kind, Purely Elizabeth)
- [ ] 1 package whole grain 6-inch tortillas
- [ ] 1 8 oz. box lentil or chickpea pasta (i.e., rotini, penne, or farfalle)
- [ ] 1 package quinoa
- [ ] 1 box whole grain crackers (i.e., Mary's Gone, Wasa, Flackers, Simple Mill)
- [ ] Gluten-free all-purpose flour
- [ ] Gluten-free panko breadcrumbs

Miscellaneous

- [ ] Coconut aminos
- [ ] Red wine vinegar
- [ ] Distilled white vinegar

- ☐ 2 quarts vegetable stock
- ☐ 1 quart chicken stock
- ☐ Sweet pickle relish
- ☐ Avocado mayonnaise (i.e., Primal Kitchen)
- ☐ Dijon mustard
- ☐ 1 small container hummus
- ☐ Miso paste
- ☐ Buffalo sauce (i.e., Primal Kitchen or Noble Made Medium Buffalo Sauce)
- ☐ Unsweetened BBQ sauce (i.e., Primal Kitchen)
- ☐ 1 bag almond flour
- ☐ Honey
- ☐ Carob chips

Dried Herbs and Spices

- ☐ Dried rosemary
- ☐ Dried oregano
- ☐ Dried thyme
- ☐ Dried basil
- ☐ Garlic powder
- ☐ Onion powder
- ☐ Sweet paprika
- ☐ Chili powder
- ☐ Ground cumin

- ☐ Bay leaf
- ☐ Black pepper
- ☐ Red pepper
- ☐ Cayenne pepper
- ☐ Salt
- ☐ Pumpkin spice
- ☐ Cinnamon

RECIPES

BREAKFAST

Egg Muffins and Fruit

Makes 6 Servings

- 2 cups chopped spinach or kale
- 1/4 cup red bell pepper, diced
- 1/4 cup mushrooms, diced
- 1/4 cup yellow onion, diced
- 1 teaspoon combination of dried rosemary, oregano, and thyme
- Salt and pepper to taste
- 12 eggs, beaten
- Olive oil or avocado oil cooking spray

Preheat oven to 375°F.

1. Mix together the vegetables, combination seasoning, sea salt, and eggs in a large bowl and then set aside.

2. Grease a 12-cup muffin pan with oil and pour the egg mix into the pan, evenly dividing among the cups.

3. Bake for about 20–25 minutes or until edges are golden brown.

4. Store in an airtight container in the refrigerator for 3–4 days. You can also freeze leftovers in a freezer-safe ziplock bag for up to three months. Thaw overnight in the refrigerator and then microwave in the morning for a quick breakfast on the go.

You can experiment with your favorite vegetable (broccoli, asparagus, tomato) and protein (turkey bacon, chicken sausage, part-skim mozzarella) combos.

You can also sauté the vegetables before assembling for extra flavor.

Raspberry Yogurt Smoothie

Makes 1 Serving

- 2/3 cup plain Greek yogurt or non-dairy yogurt
- 2/3 cup unsweetened non-dairy milk
  (i.e., almond, coconut, oat, hempseed)
- 2/3 cup frozen raspberries
- 1 tablespoon chia seeds or flaxseeds
- 1 teaspoon honey (optional)

Combine all ingredients in the jar of a blender, blend, and enjoy!

Pumpkin Spice Overnight Oats
Makes 1 Serving

- 1/3 cup old-fashioned rolled oats
- 1/3 cup unsweetened vanilla almond milk or
  non-dairy milk
- 1/4 cup pumpkin puree
- 1 tablespoon ground flaxseeds
- 1 tablespoon chia seeds
- 1/2 teaspoon pumpkin spice blend
- 1/2 teaspoon cinnamon

Optional Toppings:
- Apples or banana slices

- Pumpkin seeds or almond slivers

- Peanut butter or almond butter

- Cinnamon or pumpkin spice

1. Place oats, almond milk, pumpkin puree, flaxseeds, chia seeds, pumpkin spice blend, and cinnamon in a mason jar. Mix thoroughly to combine.

2. Cover and refrigerate overnight.

3. Add optional toppings and enjoy!

Avocado Toast and Scrambled Egg
Makes 1 Serving

- 1/3 avocado

- 2 teaspoons olive oil, divided

- 1 teaspoon lemon juice

- Salt and red pepper flakes to taste

- 1 slice sprouted grain or sourdough bread, toasted

- 2 eggs (or 1/2 cup egg whites)

- 1 oz. cheddar cheese (optional)

1. Mash the avocado in a bowl with 1 teaspoon olive oil, 1 teaspoon lemon juice, salt, and red pepper flakes. Spread the mash evenly on a piece of toasted bread.

2. Heat 1 teaspoon olive oil in a small skillet over medium heat. Whisk together the eggs and pour over the hot skillet. As the eggs begin to set, mix in the cheese, if using, and cook until melted.

3. Pour egg mixture over the avocado toast and enjoy with berries on the side.

Vegetable Omelet

Makes 1 Serving

- 2 eggs (or 1 egg and 2 egg whites)
- 1 tablespoon ghee or grass-fed butter, divided
- 1/4 cup diced multicolored bell peppers
- 1/4 cup mushrooms, sliced
- 1/4 cup medium tomatoes, diced
- 2 tablespoons cheddar cheese or vegan cream cheese
- 1 tablespoon fresh chives

1. In a small mixing bowl, whisk the eggs until they become frothy.

2. Heat a small nonstick pan over medium heat. Add 1/2 tablespoon of the ghee/butter and allow to foam.

3. Sauté the vegetables until they are lightly cooked. Remove from the pan and set on a plate.

4. Add the remaining ghee/butter to the pan. Once it melts, add the whisked eggs, stirring until they start to set.

5. Once the eggs start to set, sprinkle your sautéed vegetables and cheese in the middle of the omelet.

6. Fold the omelet in half and transfer to a plate.

Blueberry Overnight Oats
Makes 1 Serving

- 1/2 cup oats

- 1/2 cup frozen wild blueberries

- 1/2 cup unsweetened vanilla almond milk or non-dairy milk

- 1/2 cup unsweetened vanilla yogurt, Greek yogurt, or low-fat cottage cheese

- 1 tablespoon healthy fat (i.e., flaxseed, walnuts, chia seeds, almond slivers)

1. Add oatmeal to a bowl with frozen blueberries and milk and let soak overnight. (You can also skip this step and just cook the oatmeal, milk, and berries together in the morning.)

2. Stir in the yogurt or cottage cheese.

3. Top with a healthy fat and enjoy.

Note if you have a nut allergy, substitute with oat milk and top with flaxseeds.

Berry Parfait

Makes 1 Serving

- 1 individual container low-fat Greek yogurt
- 1/2 cup frozen raspberries
- 1/2 cup frozen blueberries
- 1/2 cup granola

Layer yogurt, berries, and granola in a tall glass and serve. Experiment with your favorite fruits!

LUNCH

Strawberry Chicken and Arugula Salad

Makes 4 Servings

- 4 boneless, skinless chicken breast halves (or use leftover chicken or prepared roast chicken for convenience)
- 4 sliced strawberries
- 6 cups arugula
- 2 tablespoons raw walnuts

Vinaigrette Dressing:

- 3/4 cup extra-virgin olive oil

- 1/4 cup red wine vinegar

- 2 tablespoons lemon juice

- 1 teaspoon garlic powder

- 1 teaspoon onion powder

- 1/2 teaspoon dried oregano

- 1 teaspoon dried basil

- 1/2 teaspoon sweet paprika

- Salt and pepper to taste

- 1/2 to 1 teaspoon granulated sugar, or more, to taste (optional)

1. Combine the ingredients for the dressing in a small bowl, whisk, and set aside.

2. Grill the chicken breast for 3–5 minutes on each side, or until the internal temperature reaches 165 degrees. Let cool and dice.

3. Combine the chicken, strawberries, arugula, and walnuts in a bowl.

4. Divide the salad into four servings and top each with 1–2 tablespoons of dressing. Store extra dressing in an airtight container in your refrigerator to use throughout the week.

Tuna Salad Platter
Makes 2 Servings

Salad:

- 1 (6 oz.) can water-packed tuna

- 2 tablespoons red bell pepper, diced

- 2 tablespoons yellow bell pepper, diced

- 2 tablespoons red onion, diced

- 2 tablespoons sweet pickle relish

- 2 tablespoons avocado mayonnaise (i.e., Primal Kitchen)

- 1/2 teaspoon Dijon mustard

- Sea salt and black pepper to taste

- 4 Boston lettuce leaves

- 1 tomato, sliced

- 2 cups melons

- 2/3 cup cottage cheese

1. Combine the tuna, peppers, onion, relish, mayonnaise, Dijon, salt, and pepper in a bowl. Mix well and refrigerate. Place 1/2 cup tuna salad on two Boston lettuce leaves and two tomato slices.

2. Serve each serving with 1 cup fruit and 1/3 cup cottage cheese.

Turkey Apple Wrap
Makes 6 Servings

- 1/2 pound deli-sliced turkey breast (or use leftover roast turkey)
- 1 tablespoon red onion, minced
- 1/4 cup chopped celery
- 1/4 cup chopped green apple
- 1 tablespoon dried cranberries, minced
- 1/4 teaspoon garlic granules
- 3 tablespoons avocado mayonnaise (i.e., Primal Kitchen)
- 1 tablespoon Greek yogurt
- 1/2 teaspoon Dijon mustard
- 1 tablespoon distilled white vinegar
- Pinch of dried thyme
- Pinch of sea salt
- Pinch of ground black pepper
- 6 10-inch whole-wheat or sprouted grain tortillas
- 1 1/2 cups spinach

1. Combine all ingredients except the tortillas and spinach in a large bowl and mix well.

2. Place the turkey mixture in the food processor and pulse for 2 to 3 seconds at a time until mixture is

finely diced. Alternatively, make sure the vegetables are cut into a small mince.

3. Lay the tortillas on a flat surface. Spread 1/4 cup spinach on each. Place 1/4 cup turkey mixture on top of the spinach. Roll up burrito style.

Miso Soup
Makes 4 Servings

- 1 tablespoon sesame oil
- 1/2 cup cremini mushrooms, thinly sliced
- 1/3 cup shallots, minced
- 1 quart vegetable stock
- 1 cup water
- 1/4 cup firm tofu, diced
- 3 tablespoons miso paste
- 3 tablespoons scallions, sliced
- Pinch of salt and pepper to taste

1. In a medium saucepan, heat sesame oil and cook the mushrooms. Add in shallots and cook until translucent.

2. Deglaze with vegetable stock and water, then bring to a boil. Simmer for 5 minutes. Add miso paste and tofu to heat through.

3. Place miso soup in four bowls and top with scallions. Season with salt and pepper to taste. Serve with a mixed greens side salad and Vinaigrette Dressing.

Kale Walnut Pesto Pasta Salad
Makes 4 Servings

For main dish:

- 1 (8 oz.) box lentil or chickpea pasta (rotini, penne, or farfalle)
- 1 pint cherry tomatoes, halved or quartered
- 4 handfuls baby spinach or arugula

For the kale pesto:

- 1 small bunch kale, tough ribs removed
- 1 clove garlic, peeled
- 1 cup packed fresh basil leaves
- 1/2 cup Parmesan cheese, grated
- 1/4 cup walnuts, toasted
- 1/2 cup extra-virgin olive oil
- Sea salt and pepper to taste

1. Bring a large pot of water to a boil and add a generous pinch of salt. Keep at a low boil until ready to use.

2. To make the kale pesto, blanch the kale leaves in the boiling water for 2 minutes. Using a skimmer, transfer the kale to a colander and rinse with cold water.

3. With the food processor running, drop the clove of garlic in through the top opening and process until finely minced.

4. Squeeze the blanched kale leaves to remove as much moisture as possible, and rough chop the leaves. Add to the food processor along with the basil, Parmesan cheese, and walnuts.

5. Process until the ingredients are finely chopped.

6. With the processor running, slowly drizzle in the oil and process until you have a mostly smooth paste. Season with salt and pepper to taste.

7. Cook the pasta until al dente according to package directions. Before draining, reserve about 1/2 cup pasta cooking water, then drain and immediately rinse the pasta under cool water to prevent the noodles from sticking together.

8. Transfer the cooked pasta to a serving bowl and toss with just enough kale pesto to thoroughly coat, adding a tiny splash of reserved pasta cooking water if necessary to thin it out.

9. Add the cherry tomatoes and greens.

10. Refrigerate for two hours or overnight.

Portobello Turkey Burgers

Makes 4 Servings

- 2 tablespoons avocado oil, divided
- 1/2 cup yellow onion, diced

- 2 cloves garlic, minced

- 1 pound ground turkey breast

- 1 tablespoon finely chopped parsley

- Salt and pepper to taste

- 8 portobello mushrooms, washed and stems removed

- 1 tomato, sliced

- 4 Boston lettuce leaves

1. In a small sauté pan, sauté onions in 1 tablespoon of avocado oil until translucent/soft. Add garlic for the last minute of cooking. Let cool.

2. In a large mixing bowl, combine the ground turkey breast, onions, garlic, parsley, salt, and pepper.

3. Shape into 4 burgers. Place on a plate in the refrigerator for 30 minutes to set.

4. Rub the rest of the avocado oil on the portobello mushrooms and season with salt and pepper on both sides.

5. Heat a grill and cook the portobello mushroom slices and turkey burgers until the internal temperature of the burgers reaches 165 degrees.

6. Serve each turkey burger between two portobello mushroom slices, topped with tomato, lettuce, and your favorite condiments. Serve with a mixed greens side salad and Vinaigrette Dressing.

Simple Lentil Soup

Makes 4 Servings

- 2 tablespoons olive oil

- 1 small yellow onion, minced

- 2 carrots, minced

- 2 celery stalks, minced

- 1 cup red lentils, rinsed

- 1 cup diced tomatoes with juices

- 4 cups vegetable broth

- 2 cups filtered water

- 1 bay leaf

- 2 cups kale or spinach, chopped

- 1 tablespoon Dijon mustard

- 1 tablespoon red wine vinegar

- Salt and pepper to taste

1. Heat a Dutch oven or large pot over medium heat and coat the bottom of the pot with olive oil.

2. Sauté the onions, carrots, and celery until the onions are translucent and vegetables are cooked through.

3. Add the lentils to lightly toast, followed by the tomatoes with juices.

4. Add the vegetable broth and filtered water.

5. Bring to a boil, reduce heat, and simmer for 30 minutes.

6. Wilt in the greens and simmer a few more minutes.

7. Stir in the Dijon mustard and red wine vinegar.

8. Season with salt and pepper to taste. Serve with a slice of sourdough bread or sprouted grain bread.

DINNER

One-Pot Shrimp Scampi and Broccoli
Makes 4 Servings

- 1 pound large shrimp, peeled and deveined
- 3 tablespoons extra-virgin olive oil, divided
- 1 tablespoon lemon zest, plus 1 tablespoon juice (from 1 lemon)
- 1/2 teaspoon red pepper flakes
- Salt and black pepper to taste
- 4 garlic cloves, minced and divided
- 2 tablespoons unsalted butter
- 1 cup orzo
- 1/3 cup dry white wine (or substitute with chicken stock)
- 2 cups chicken stock

- 2 cups broccoli florets, stems removed
- 1/2 cup Parmesan cheese, shredded
- 2 tablespoons finely chopped parsley

1. In a medium bowl, stir together shrimp, 1 tablespoon olive oil, lemon zest, red pepper flakes, salt, pepper, and half the garlic. Set aside to marinate for 20–30 minutes.

2. Heat a medium brassier or larger skillet set over medium heat. Add the butter, remaining olive oil, and remaining garlic. When the butter starts to bubble, add the orzo and a dash of salt, and toast the orzo, stirring often, about 2 minutes. Turn the heat to low to add the wine and stir until absorbed, about 1 minute. Stir in the chicken broth and cover the pot. Simmer the orzo until al dente, about 12 minutes.

3. Add the shrimp and broccoli in a snug, even layer on top of the orzo, cover, and cook until all the shrimp is pink and cooked through, approximately 5 minutes. Remove from heat and let sit, covered, 2 minutes.

4. Mix in the Parmesan cheese and lemon juice, then season with salt and pepper. Sprinkle with parsley and serve immediately.

Buffalo Turkey Chili and
Almond Coconut Drop Biscuits

Makes 6 Servings

- 1 tablespoon olive oil

- 2 pounds ground turkey breast (or ground chicken breast)

- 2 large carrots, peeled and cut into large dice

- 2 stalks celery, large dice

- 1 large red bell pepper, large dice

- 4 cloves garlic

- 1 tablespoon chili powder

- 1 tablespoon ground cumin

- 1/2 tablespoon paprika

- 1/2 cup buffalo sauce
  (i.e., Primal Kitchen or Noble Made
  Medium Buffalo Sauce)

- 1 (15 oz.) can tomato sauce

- 1 (15 oz.) can diced tomatoes

- 1 (15 oz.) can chili beans in sauce (do not drain)

- Salt and pepper to taste

1. Heat a heavy pot over medium heat and add the oil. Cook the turkey breast, breaking it up with a spoon, until no longer pink.

2. While the turkey is cooking, prepare the vegetables. Place the carrots, celery, bell pepper, and garlic in a clean food processor bowl and puree. Alternatively, cut the vegetables into a small mince.

3. Add the vegetable mixture to the pot with the cooked turkey and cook until the vegetables start to soften, about 5 minutes.

4. Stir in the chili powder, cumin, paprika, buffalo sauce, tomato sauce, diced tomatoes, and chili beans with their sauce. Season with salt and pepper to taste.

5. Bring to a boil and reduce the heat to a simmer. Cook for 1 hour.

6. Season with additional salt and pepper to taste and serve with your favorite garnishes and 1 Almond Coconut Drop Biscuit.

Almond Coconut Drop Biscuits

Makes 8 Servings

- 2 tablespoons coconut butter, cubed
- 2 tablespoons coconut oil, solid
- 2 1/2 cups almond flour
- 1 tablespoon baking powder
- 1/2 teaspoon Himalayan pink salt

- 3/4 cup plain unsweetened Greek yogurt or non-dairy yogurt

- 1 large egg, beaten

1. Preheat the oven to 350°F. Line a baking sheet with parchment paper.

2. Combine the coconut butter and coconut oil in a small bowl and chill in the freezer for about 5 minutes.

3. In a medium mixing bowl or food processor, whisk together the flour, baking powder, and salt. Add the chilled coconut butter and coconut oil and cut in using a pastry blender if doing by hand, until a meal forms. Add in the yogurt and form the dough into a ball.

4. Use an ice cream scoop to make 8 drop biscuits and place on the parchment-lined baking sheet.

5. Using a pastry brush, lightly coat the top of each biscuit with the beaten egg (optional).

6. Bake for approximately 20 minutes until golden brown.

**Salmon with Soy Glaze
and Roasted Asparagus**

Makes 4 Servings

- 2 6-oz. portions of wild salmon (ask for it deboned but with skin on)

- 1 teaspoon Dijon mustard

- 1 tablespoon coconut aminos

- 1 teaspoon avocado oil, plus more as needed

- 1 clove garlic, minced

1. Preheat the broiler on high with the top rack about 4 inches from the top.

2. Mix marinade for salmon in a small bowl: Dijon, coconut aminos, avocado oil, and minced garlic. On a foil-lined sheet tray, drizzle a teeny bit of avocado oil to keep the salmon from sticking, and then place salmon skin side down. Spoon the marinade evenly over the salmon. Clean up any excess oil or marinade on the foil with a paper towel to avoid smoking in the oven. Let sit for 2–10 minutes.

3. Place the salmon under the broiler and cook for 3–5 minutes. Keep an eye on this until you get used to your broiler. The marinade should form a nice glaze on top and the salmon should cook through while staying pink in the middle. If salmon starts to burn, the broiler is too hot—turn off the broiler

and turn on the oven to 400°F and finish cooking. If you are using a thermometer, aim for an internal temperature of 120°F.

4. Serve with roasted asparagus.

Roasted Asparagus

Makes 4 Servings

•   1 pound asparagus

•   2 tablespoons olive oil

•   Salt and red pepper flakes to taste

1. Preheat oven to 400°F.

2. Line a baking sheet with parchment paper or a baking mat.

3. Toss asparagus with olive oil, salt, and red pepper flakes. Space them out so the asparagus are not touching.

4. Roast for 10–12 minutes.

Black Bean and Quinoa Burger
with Carrot and Green Bean Fries
Makes 6 Servings

- 2 tablespoons extra-virgin olive oil

- 1 onion, medium dice

- 1/2 cup quinoa

- 1 cup water

- 1 cup black beans, drained and rinsed

- 1 1/2 tablespoons coconut aminos

- 3/4 cup walnuts

- 2 cloves garlic, minced

- 1/2 cup fresh cilantro, packed

- 3/4 teaspoon ground cumin

- 1/4 teaspoon cayenne pepper

- Salt and pepper to taste

- 1/4 cup gluten-free all-purpose flour

- 1 cup gluten-free panko breadcrumbs

- 2 eggs, lightly beaten

- 2 cups arugula

- Lemon juice and extra-virgin olive oil to taste

1. Heat a saucepan over medium heat and add the olive oil. Gently sauté the onion until lightly caramelized around the edges, 5 to 6 minutes. Stir in the quinoa and toast for 1 minute.

2. Add the water, bring to a boil, and then lower the heat to a simmer. Cook, covered, until the water has absorbed, 18 to 20 minutes. Remove from the heat and rest, covered, for 10 minutes.

3. Place the cooked quinoa in a food processor and add the black beans, coconut aminos, walnuts, garlic, cilantro, cumin, and cayenne. Process until finely chopped. Season with salt and pepper. Transfer to a mixing bowl and fold in the flour, panko, and eggs.

4. Form rounded 1/2 cups of mixture into six (3 1/2-inch diameter) patties and set them on a parchment-lined tray. Chill at least 10 minutes. (Patties may be individually wrapped and frozen at this point.)

5. Heat a griddle over medium heat and brush with avocado oil. Place the burgers on the hot griddle and cook until browned and crisp on the outside and warm all the way through, about 5 minutes per side.

6. While the burgers are cooking, toss the arugula with the lemon juice and olive oil, then season with salt and pepper.

7. Serve with arugula salad and vegetables fries.

Carrot and Green Bean Fries
Makes 6 Servings

- 2 cups carrots, cut into fry shapes similar to the green beans in size
- 2 cups whole green beans
- 1 1/2 teaspoons extra-virgin olive oil
- 1/4 teaspoon sea salt
- 1/4 teaspoon freshly ground black pepper

1. Preheat the broiler. Line a baking sheet with aluminum foil. In a large bowl, toss the carrots, green beans, oil, salt, and pepper.

2. Spread the carrots and green beans in a single layer on the prepared baking sheet.

3. Broil for about 7 minutes, turning once halfway through the cooking time. These are best right out of the oven.

Baked Fish in Parchment Paper and Greek Lemon Potatoes
Makes 4 Servings

- 4 16-inch parchment paper sheets
- 4 fresh rosemary sprigs
- 4 white fish filets (4–6 oz.)

- 1 cup zucchini, diced

- 8 cherry tomatoes, halved

- 4 small artichoke hearts (canned), halved

- 2 tablespoons avocado or grapeseed oil

- Salt and pepper to taste

- 1 lemon, juiced

1. Preheat oven to 425°F.

2. Lay rosemary sprigs at the bottom of the parchment paper. Season the fish filets with salt and pepper. Place them on top of the rosemary, in the middle of the parchment paper.

3. In a medium bowl, toss zucchini, tomatoes, and artichokes with salt, pepper, and avocado oil. Evenly divide over each filet.

4. Seal the packet by rolling and crimping the long sides together over the fish and vegetables. Then roll and crimp the end so no steam can escape. Place packets on a baking sheet.

5. Bake for approximately 12–15 minutes until the fish are cooked through. Note that 1/2-inch filets will finish quicker than 1 inch.

6. Carefully open the packets as steam will escape. Top with lemon juice and serve with potatoes.

Greek Lemon Potatoes
Makes 4–6 Servings

- 3 medium-size russet potatoes, washed and cut into 1-inch wedges
- 2 tablespoons extra-virgin olive oil
- 1 teaspoon dried oregano
- Salt and pepper to taste
- Lemon juice to taste
- 1/3 cup feta cheese, crumbled (optional)

1. Preheat the oven to 400°F.

2. Place the potatoes on a baking sheet and toss with the olive oil and oregano.

3. Season with salt and pepper to taste.

4. Roast the potatoes until tender and golden brown around the edges, 35 to 40 minutes.

5. Transfer the hot potatoes to a platter and top with a squeeze of fresh lemon juice.

6. Top with a sprinkling of feta cheese (optional).

BBQ Sheet Tray Chicken Dinner
Makes 4 Servings

- 4 boneless, skinless chicken breasts
- 2 cups brussels sprouts, cleaned and sliced in half

- 4 sweet potatoes, sliced into wedges
- 1/2 cup unsweetened BBQ sauce, divided
- 2 tablespoons avocado oil, divided
- 1/4 teaspoon chili powder
- Salt and pepper to taste

1. Preheat oven to 425°F and line a rimmed baking sheet with parchment paper or a baking mat.

2. Brush both sides of each chicken breast using half of the BBQ sauce. Place to one side of the baking sheet.

3. Drizzle the potatoes with 1 tablespoon of oil and sprinkle with chili powder and salt. Use tongs to toss the potatoes so each piece is evenly coated, and place in the middle of the baking sheet.

4. Drizzle the brussels sprouts with 1 tablespoon of oil and sprinkle with salt and pepper. Use tongs to toss the sprouts so each piece is evenly coated then place on the other side of the baking sheet.

5. Place the baking sheet in the oven and roast until the chicken is completely cooked through and reads an internal temperature of 160°F and the brussels sprouts and potato wedges are tender and charred in spots, approximately 25 minutes.

6. Brush chicken with remaining BBQ sauce before serving.

Note that you may flip chicken breasts and potato wedges halfway through for more even cooking.

SNACKS

Beauty Protein Bites
Makes 12 Servings (24 protein balls)

- 1/2 cup unsweetened cashew butter

- 1/4 cup mini carob chips or dark chocolate nibs

- 1 cup old-fashioned oats (gluten-free)

- 2 tablespoons ground flaxseeds

- 2 tablespoons walnuts, chopped

- 1/4 cup honey

- 1 teaspoon cinnamon

- Dash of salt

1. Stir all the ingredients together in a large bowl.

2. Place the bowl in the refrigerator for 15 minutes so the mixture becomes firmer and easier to scoop into a ball.

3. Use a tablespoon cookie scoop (or spoon) and form the mixture into balls by rolling the mixture with your hands. Place balls on a cookie sheet to set.

4. Store in the refrigerator for 1 week in an airtight container or freeze for up to one month by wrapping two bites together (one serving) in plastic wrap and then placing the servings into a freezer bag.

**Roasted Kale
and Pumpkin Seed Chips**
Makes 2 Servings

- 1 bunch kale, chopped with stems removed

- 1 tablespoon olive oil

- 1 tablespoon pumpkin seeds

- 1/4 teaspoon sea salt

- 1/4 teaspoon ground black pepper

1. Preheat oven to 350°F and set out a baking sheet.

2. In a large bowl toss the kale leaves with olive oil, pumpkin seeds, salt, and pepper, rubbing the leaves with your fingers to coat with the oil and spices.

3. Arrange the leaves over the baking sheet and bake for 8–10 minutes. If the leaves are not crispy in the center, bake for another few minutes.

4. Enjoy as a snack or a crispy topping for your soup or salad.

Store leftover kale chips after they are cooled in an airtight container at room temperature for 2–3 days.

Turkey Roll-Ups
Makes 1 Serving

- 2 slices of turkey
- 1 tablespoon hummus (of your choice)
- 1/3 red bell pepper, sliced thin
- 1/3 yellow bell pepper, sliced thin
- 1/3 cucumber, sliced thin

Spread hummus evenly over both slices of turkey and top each with 1/2 the bell peppers and cucumber. Roll them up and enjoy!

MOOD-BOOSTING SNACKS

Some individuals prefer to eat every four hours to keep their energy levels high and reduce cravings.

Choose a fibrous protein-rich snack from the list below when you need a mood boost:

- Apple with 1 tablespoon unsweetened almond butter, cashew butter, or peanut butter
- 1 serving fruit or non-starchy vegetables and 1 piece string cheese
- Celery sticks with 1 tablespoon unsweetened nut butter, unsweetened raisins, and cinnamon

- Apple, orange, peach, or plum and serving of almonds, walnuts halves, or cashews

- Vegetable sticks with 1/4 cup hummus

- 1 hard-boiled egg and 1 serving of fruit or non-starchy vegetables

- 1/2 cup low-fat cottage cheese and 1 cup berries or celery and carrot sticks

- 2/3 cup low-fat Greek yogurt and 1/2 cup sliced fruit

- Trail mix (1/4 cup serving)—make your own by mixing a combination of your favorite nuts, seeds, unsweetened dried fruit, and dark chocolate nibs

- 1 brown rice cake or 1 serving whole grain crackers (Mary's Gone, Wasa, Flackers, Simple Mill Almond Flour Crackers) with 1 tablespoon unsweetened almond butter, cashew butter, peanut butter, or string cheese

ACKNOWLEDGMENTS

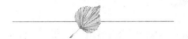

I AM DEEPLY GRATEFUL to all my family and friends for their unwavering support and encouragement. I am truly blessed in life because there are too many of you to personally acknowledge and mention.

My heartfelt thanks go to my parents, Bob and Joan Clifford. Since I was a little girl, you inspired me to dream big and love life. Dad, you are a true renaissance man, and I have always admired your passion for justice and helping others. Mom, you have the biggest heart and bring a little sparkle wherever you go.

To my husband, John Kalantzis. You are my best friend, biggest support, and an exceptional editor. I love our life together and feel fortunate every day to have you by my side.

To my sister Tracy Clifford Esbrook, who pushed

me to find my jam and pursue my passion for wellness. Dominic and Roman, my two nephews, you bring so much joy to my life. You are intelligent and creative beyond your years.

To "my big sister," Carrie Clifford. Thank you for believing in me and being a daily sounding board. You always remind me to take a breath and practice what I preach.

To my partner in crime Rachel Baker. You always help make any crazy idea that I have a reality. I could never have created this book without your guidance and steadfast friendship.

To my marketing team at Web Marketing Therapy. Lorrie Thomas Ross, you taught me how to build an authentic brand and blessed me with your friendship. Katherine Garcia, you are my biggest cheerleader and helped inspire my wellness teachings. Anne Orfila, you guided me in taking my brand to another level and have been instrumental in developing my wellness programs. Cinder Thomas, the graphics you have created brought my vision to life.

To my guru and girlfriend Loren Lahav. I can't thank you enough for your tremendous guidance and confidence in me. You taught me that success takes time and to keep being true to myself.

To my friend and mentor, Justice Terrence J. Lavin. Thank you for taking a chance on me right out of law school. You taught me how to write and shaped my confidence as a young professional. You also connected me with my lifelong girlfriends Kim Guernsey and Marya Lucas who bought me my first no button.

To the Positive Sobriety Institute, especially my supervisors Michael Geraci and Katie Sleman. Thank you for allowing me to do my clinical internship with you. Your teachings and guidance are present in these pages.

To all the faculty and students that I had the privilege of studying with at The Family Institute at Northwestern University. You inspired me throughout my schooling and pushed me to think outside the box.

To all the chefs at The Chopping Block who turned me into a talented recreational cook, especially my friend and executive chef / owner Lisa Counts. You helped shape my nutrition philosophy, which I have made an integral part of my coaching program.

To my editor and friend Ami McConnell. Thank you for helping me find my voice and emboldening me to be brave and share my story.

To my photographer and friend Michelle Nolan.

Thank you for always capturing my authentic side and your creative inspiration.

Thank you to my amazing team at Forefront Books, including Jonathan Merkh, Jill Smith, Lauren Ward, Landry Parkey, and Rebekah Guzman.

Thank you to all my individual and corporate clients for inspiring me every day. I have learned so much from you and it has been an honor to be your coach on your wellness journeys.

Finally, to my children with paws, Bella, Gatsby, and Daisy. You are my lights, and I have been truly touched by your unconditional love and companionship.

ABOUT THE AUTHOR

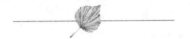

ERIN CLIFFORD helps professionals develop healthy lifestyles for a more fulfilling existence. Her wellness coaching, seminars, and programs are built on a holistic approach that includes nutrition, physical activity, sleep, stress management, mindfulness, healthy relationships, career goals, and mental health. Erin has trained with some of the world's top nutrition, diet, exercise, and wellness experts. Born and raised in Chicago, Erin began her career teaching for Chicago Public Schools and holds a Juris Doctor from DePaul College of Law. She's the managing director at Clifford Law Offices, a Licensed Professional Counselor in Illinois, and a National Certified Counselor with a master's degree in clinical mental health counseling from Northwestern University. She also holds numerous health and wellness coaching certifications and is a National Board Certified Health & Wellness Coach (NBC-HWC). You can find and follow her at erincliffordwellness.com.

NOTES

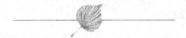

INTRODUCTION

1. "Workplace Stress," American Institute of Stress, 2024, https://www.stress.org/workplace-stress#:~:text=83%25%20of%20US%20workers%20suffer,stress%20affects%20their%20personal%20relationships.

2. Shipra Bansal, Meaghan Connolly, and Tasha Harder, "Impact of a Whole-Foods, Plant-Based Nutrition Intervention on Patients Living with Chronic Disease in an Underserved Community," *American Journal of Lifestyle Medicine* 16, no. 3 (2021): 382–89, https://doi.org/10.1177/15598276211018159.

CHAPTER 1

3. Rebekka Kesberg and Johannes Keller, "The Relation Between Human Values and Perceived Situation Characteristics in Everyday Life," *Frontiers in Psychology* 9 (2018): 1–15, https://doi.org/10.3389/fpsyg.2018.01676.

4.   Dana Paliliunas, "Values: A Core Guiding Principle for Behavior-Analytic Intervention and Research," *Behavioral Analysis in Practice* 15, no. 1 (2021): 115–25, https://doi.org/10.1007/s40617-021-00595-3.

CHAPTER 2

5.   Dan Buettner and Sam Skemp, "Blue Zones: Lessons from the World's Longest Lived American," *Journal of Lifestyle Medicine* 10, no. 5 (2016): 318–21, https://pubmed.ncbi.nlm.nih.gov/30202288/.

6.   Nicholas G. Norwitz and Uma Naidoo, "Nutrition as Metabolic Treatment for Anxiety," *Frontiers in Psychiatry* 12 (2021): 598119, https://doi.org/10.3389/fpsyt.2021.598119.

7.   Pedro Mateos-Aparicio and Antonio Rodríguez-Moreno, "The Impact of Studying Brain Plasticity," *Frontiers in Cellular Neuroscience* 13, no. 66 (2019): 1–5, https://doi.org/10.3389/fncel.2019.00066; "Mental Illness," National Institute of Mental Health (NIMH), accessed November 6, 2024, https://www.nimh.nih.gov/health/statistics/mental-illness.

8.   Nicky J. Newton, Preet K. Chauhan, and Jessica L. Pates, "Facing the Future: Generativity, Stagnation, Intended Legacies, and Well-Being in Later Life," *Journal of Adult Development* 27 (2020): 70–80, https://doi.org/10.1007/s10804-019-09330-3.

9.   Robert Emmons, Jeffrey Froh, and Rachel Rose, "Gratitude," in M. W. Gallagher and S. J. Lopez, eds., *Positive Psychological Assessment: A Handbook of Models and Measures*, American Psychological Association, 317–32, https://doi.org/10.1037/0000138-020.

CHAPTER 3

10. Ellen Ernst Kossek, "Managing Work Life Boundaries in the Digital Age," *Organizational Dynamics* 45, no. 3 (2016): 258–70. https://doi.org/10.1016/j.orgdyn.2016.07.010.

11. Helen Pluut and Jaap Wonders "Not Able to Lead a Healthy Life When You Need It the Most: Dual Role of Lifestyle Behaviors in the Association of Blurred Work-Life Boundaries with Well-Being," *Frontiers in Psychology* 11 (2020): 1–15, https://doi.org/10.3389/fpsyg.2020.607294.

12. Ariane G. Wepfer et al., "Work-Life Boundaries and Well-Being: Does Work-to-Life Integration Impair Well-Being Through Lack of Recovery?," *Journal of Business and Psychology* 33, no. 6 (2018): 727–40, https://doi.org/10.1007/s10869-017-9520-y.

CHAPTER 4

13. Barbara Riegel et al., "Self-Care Research: Where Are We Now? Where Are We Going?," *International Journal of Nursing Studies* 116 (2021): 103402, https://doi.org/10.1016/j.ijnurstu.2019.103402.

14. Christian Montag et al., "Linking Individual Differences in Satisfaction with Each of Maslow's Needs to the Big Five Personality Traits and Panksepp's Primary Emotional Systems," *Heliyon* 6, no. 7 (2020): e04325–e04325, https://doi:10.1016/j.heliyon.2020.e04325.

15. Nicole Martínez et al., "Self-Care: A Concept Analysis," *International Journal of Nursing Sciences* 8, no. 4 (2021): 418–25, https://doi.org/10.1016/j.ijnss.2021.08.007.

CHAPTER 5

16. Riegel, "Self-Care Research."

17. Katherine R. Arlinghaus and Craig A. Johnston, "The Importance of Creating Habits and Routine," *American Journal of Lifestyle Medicine* 13, no. 2 (2018): 142–44, https://doi .org/10.1177/1559827618818044.

CHAPTER 6

18. S. Brewer, *What Happened to Moderation? A Common-Sense Approach to Improving Our Health and Treating Common Illnesses in an Age of Extremes* (SelectBooks Inc., 2019).

19. Brewer and Yun Jun Yang, "An Overview of Current Physical Activity Recommendations in Primary Care," *Korean Journal of Family Medicine* 40, no. 3 (2019): 135–42, https://doi .org/10.4082/kjfm.19.0038.

20. A. A. Sayer et al., "The Developmental Origins of Sarcopenia," *The Journal of Nutrition, Health & Aging* 12, no. 7 (2008): 427–32, https://doi.org/10.1007/BF02982703.

21. Kathleen Mikkelsen et al., "Exercise and Mental Health," *Maturitas* 106 (2017): 48–56, https://doi.org/10.1016 /j.maturitas.2017.09.003.

22. Brewer and Yang, "An Overview of Current Physical Activity Recommendations in Primary Care."

23. Annalisa Geraci et al., "Sarcopenia and Menopause: The Role of Estradiol," *Frontiers in Endocrinology* 12 (2021): 1–5, https://doi .org/10.3389/fendo.2021.682012.

CHAPTER 7

24. H. Francis, and R. Stevenson, "Validity and Test-Retest Reliability of a Short Dietary Questionnaire to Assess Intake of Saturated Fat and Free Sugars: A Preliminary Study," *Journal of Human Nutrition & Dietetics* 26, no. 3 (2013): 234–42, https://doi.org/10.1111/jhn.12008.

25. J. Lee and J. Allen, "Gender Differences in Healthy and Unhealthy Food Consumption and Its Relationship With Depression in Young Adulthood," *Community Mental Health Journal,* 57, no. 5 (2021): 898–909, https://doi.org/10.1007/s10597-020-00672-x.

26. Felice N. Jacka et al., "A Randomized Controlled Trial of Dietary Improvement for Adults with Major Depression (The 'Smiles' Trial)," *BMC Medicine* 5, no. 1 (2017): 23, https://doi.org/10.1186/s12916-017-0791-y.

27. Laura LaChance and Drew Ramsey, "Antidepressant Foods: An Evidence-Based Nutrient Profiling System for Depression," *World Journal of Psychiatry* 8, no. 3 (2018): 97–104, https://doi.org/10.5498/wjp.v8.i3.97.

28. Rachel Freire, "Scientific Evidence of Diets for Weight Loss: Different Macronutrient Composition, Intermittent Fasting, and Popular Diets," *Nutrition* 69 (2020): 110549, https://doi.org/10.1016/j.nut.2019.07.001.

29. Peter Attia, *Outlive: The Science & Art of Longevity* (Harmony Books, 2023).

30. Harvard T. H. Chan School of Public Health, "Fruits and Vegetables," The Nutrition Source, accessed November 7, 2024, https://www.hsph.harvard.edu/nutritionsource/what-should-you-eat/vegetables-and-fruits/.

31. LaChance and Ramsey, "Antidepressant Foods."

32. J. J. Virgin, *The Virgin Diet* (HarperCollins, 2012).

33. Freydis Hjalmarsdottir, "17 Science-Based Benefits of Omega-3 Fatty Acids," Healthline.com, January 17, 2023, https://www.healthline.com/nutrition/17-health-benefits-of-omega-3#TOC_TITLE_HDR_14.

34. Kris Gunnars, "Are Vegetable and Seed Oils Bad for Your Health?," Healthline.com, updated June 9, 2023, https://www.healthline.com/nutrition/are-vegetable-and-seed-oils-bad.

35. Mayo Clinic Staff, "Water: How Much Should You Drink Every Day?," Mayoclinic.org, October 12, 2022, https://www.mayoclinic.org/healthy-lifestyle/nutrition-and-healthy-eating/in-depth/water/art-20044256.

36. D. G. Smith, "Even a Little Alcohol Can Harm Your Health," *New York Times*, January 13, 2023, https://www.nytimes.com/2023/01/13/well/mind/alcohol-health-effects.html.

37. Anthony Winston, Elizabeth Hardwick, and Neema Jaberi, "Neuropsychiatric Effects of Caffeine," *Advances in Psychiatric Treatment* 11, no. 6 (2005): 432–39, https://doi.org/10.1192/apt.11.6.432.

CHAPTER 8

38. "Workplace Stress," American Institute of Stress.

39. S. M. Southwick et al., "Resilience: An Update. PTSD," *Research Quarterly* 25, no. 4 (2015): 1050–835.

40. Jenna E. Boyd, Ruth A. Lanius, and Margaret C. McKinnon, "Mindfulness-Based Treatments for Posttraumatic Stress Disorder: A Review of the Treatment Literature and Neurobiological Evidence," *Journal of Psychiatry and Neuroscience* 43, no. 1 (2018):

7–25, https://doi.org/10.1503/jpn.170021.

41. James N. Donald et al., "Daily Stress and the Benefits of Mindfulness: Examining the Daily and Longitudinal Relations Between Present-Moment Awareness and Stress Responses," *Journal of Research in Personality* 65 (2016): 30–37, http://dx.doi.org/10.1016/j.jrp.2016.09.002.

42. Boyd, Lanius, and McKinnon, "Mindfulness-Based Treatments for Posttraumatic Stress Disorder."

43. Lauren R. Locklear, Sharon Sheridan, and Dejun Tony Kong, "Appreciating Social Science Research on Gratitude: An Integrative Review for Organizational Scholarship on Gratitude in the Workplace," *Journal of Organizational Behavior* 44, no. 2 (2023): 225–60, https://doi.org/10.1002/job.2624.

CHAPTER 9

44. Max Hirshkowitz et al., "National Sleep Foundation's Sleep Time Duration Recommendations: Methodology and Results Summary," *Sleep Health* 1, no. 1 (2015): 40–43, https://doi.org/10.1016/j.sleh.2014.12.010.

45. Susan L. Worley, "The Extraordinary Importance of Sleep: The Detrimental Effects of Inadequate Sleep on Health and Public Safety Drive an Explosion of Sleep Research," *Pharmacy & Therapeutics* 43, no. 12 (2018): 758–63, https://www.ncbi.nlm.nih.gov/pmc/articles/PMC6281147/.

46. Kannan Ramar et al., "Sleep Is Essential to Health: An American Academy of Sleep Medicine Position Statement," *Journal of Clinical Sleep Medicine* 17, no. 10 (2021): 2115–119, https://doi.org/10.5664/jcsm.9476.

47. Ramar et al., "Sleep Is Essential to Health."

Notes

48. M. G. Figueiro et al., "The Impact of Daytime Light Exposures on Sleep and Mood in Office Workers," *Sleep Health* 3, no. 3 (2017): 204–15, https://doi.org/10.1016/j.sleh.2017.03.005.

49. Anthony Winston, Elizabeth Hardwick, and Neema Jaberi, "Neuropsychiatric Effects of Caffeine," *Advances in Psychiatric Treatment* 11, no. 6 (2005): 432–39, https://doi.org/10.1192/apt.11.6.432.

50. "Exercising for Better Sleep," Johns Hopkins Medicine, August 8, 2021, https://www.hopkinsmedicine.org/health/wellness-and-prevention/exercising-for-better-sleep.

51. Smith, "Even a Little Alcohol Can Harm Your Health."

52. Marcia Ines Silvani et al., "The Influence of Blue Light on Sleep, Performance and Wellbeing in Young Adults: A Systematic Review," *Frontiers in Physiology*, no. 13 (2022): 943108, https://doi.org/10.3389/fphys.2022.943108.

53. Yeonsu Kim et al., "The Impact of Forced Awakening on Morning Blood Pressure Surge," *Heart & Lung*, no. 68 (2024): 92–97, https://doi.org/10.1016/j.hrtlng.2024.06.011.

CHAPTER 10

54. Osahon Ogbeiwi, "Why Written Objectives Need to Be Really SMART," *British Journal of Healthcare Management* 23 (2017): 324–36, https://doi.org/10.12968/bjhc.2017.23.7.324.

55. H. J. Klein et al., "When Goals Are Known: The Effects of Audience Relative Status on Goal Commitment and Performance," *Journal of Applied Psychology* 105, no. 4 (2020): 372–89, https://doi.org/10.1037/apl0000441.

CHAPTER 11

56. W. Yin et al., "Mediterranean Diet and Depression: A Population-Based Cohort Study," *The International Journal of Behavioral Nutrition and Physical Activity 18, no. 1 (2021):* 1–153. https://doi .org/10.1186/s12966-021-01227-3.

57. J. Santos Vaz et al., "Dietary Patterns, N-3 Fatty Acids Intake from Seafood and High Levels of Anxiety Symptoms During Pregnancy: Findings from the Avon Longitudinal Study of Parents and Children," *PLOS One* 8, no. 7 (2013): e67671, https://doi .org/10.1371/journal.pone.0067671.

58. LaChance and Ramsey, "Antidepressant Foods."

59. Carisha S. Thesing et al., "Omega-3 and Omega-6 Fatty Acid Levels in Depressive and Anxiety Disorders," *Psychoneuroendocrinology* 87 (2018): 53–62, https://doi.org/10.1016/j.psyneuen.2017.10.005.

60. Matthew R. Hilimire, Jordan E. DeVylder, and Catherine A. Forestell, "Fermented Food, Neuroticism, and Social Anxiety: An Interaction Model," *Psychiatry Research* 228, no. 2 (2015): 203–8, https://doi.org/10.1016/j.psychres.2015.04.023.

61. Ingvar Bjelland et al., "Choline in Anxiety and Depression: The Hordaland Health Study," *The American Journal of Clinical Nutrition* 90, no. 4 (2009): 1056–60, https://doi.org/10.3945 /ajcn.2009.27493.

62. G. Addolorato et al., "Anxiety but Not Depression Decreases in Celiac Patients After One-Year Gluten-Free Diet," *Digestive and Liver Disease* 32, no. 2 (2000): 113, https://doi.org/10.1016 /S1590-8658(00)80627-1.

63. Anthony Winston, Elizabeth Hardwick, and Neema Jaberi, "Neuropsychiatric Effects of Caffeine," *Advances in Psychiatric Treatment* 11, no. 6 (2005): 432–39, https://doi.org/10.1192 /apt.11.6.432.

CONCLUSION

64. A. A. Tseng, "Scientific Evidence of Health Benefits by Practicing Mantra Meditation: Narrative Review," *International Journal of Yoga* 15, no. 2 (2022): 89–95, https://doi.org/10.4103/ijoy. ijoy_53_22.